DOC, FIX MY PLATE!

DOC, FIX MY PLATE!

The Physician In the Kitchen®'s Prescriptions for Your Healthy Meal Makeover

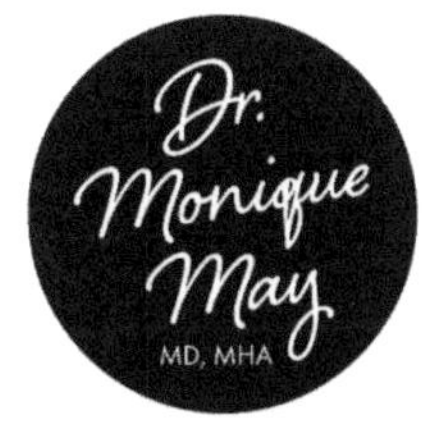

Foreword By Tedd and Hazel May

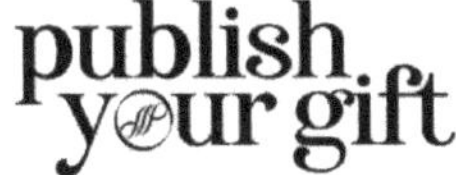

DOC, FIX MY PLATE!

Copyright © 2022 Monique May
All rights reserved.

Published by Publish Your Gift
An imprint of Purposely Created Publishing Group, LLC

No part of this book may be reproduced, distributed or transmitted in any form by any means, graphic, electronic, or mechanical, including photocopy, recording, taping, or by any information storage or retrieval system, without permission in writing from the publisher, except in the case of reprints in the context of reviews, quotes, or references.

The information in this book is not meant to prevent, diagnose, treat or cure any disease. This book is not intended as a substitute for the medical advice of your personal physician. The reader should regularly consult a physician in matters relating to one's health and particularly with respect to any symptoms that may require diagnosis or medical attention.

Unless otherwise indicated, scripture quotations are from the Holy Bible, King James Version. All rights reserved.

Printed in the United States of America

ISBN: 978-1-64484-544-8 (print)
ISBN: 978-1-64484-545-5 (ebook)

Special discounts are available on bulk quantity purchases by book clubs, associations and special interest groups. For details email: sales@publishyourgift.com or call (888) 949-6228.
For information log on to www.PublishYourGift.com

"O taste and see that the Lord is good."

—Psalm 34:8

"When diet is wrong, medicine is of no use. When diet is correct, medicine is of no need."

—Ayurvedic proverb

"He loved the GOTS: Goodies On The Stove!"

—Mommy

"I feel full. . . . and healthy!"

—Kimberly A.

"Don't count the days. Make the days count."

—Muhammad Ali

To Daddy and Mommy

Look what you started when you bought me that little Easy-Bake Oven all those years ago! Thank you for always loving me, supporting me, and being my first taste testers!

To Mitchell Ellis

You are the inspiration for everything I do, especially since you told me you needed to eat "something you put on a plate." Thanks for being a good sport and at least trying my vegan creations, even when you knew I was trying to pull one over on you.

To Rob

Thank you for sharing
My love of food, for being
My sounding board too.

To my besties, Kim, Dagmar, and Natasha

Thank you for being the sisters I never had! Thank you for also serving as taste testers and some of my very first customers. Your love and support mean more than you will ever know!

THANK YOU

for purchasing my book!

Go to rxhealthyplate.com

and subscribe to get your

FREE GIFT!

Table of Contents

FOREWORD XV

INTRODUCTION 1

CHAPTER 1: VEGAN BASICS 101 3

CHAPTER 2 SETTING UP THE VEGAN PANTRY 19

CHAPTER 3: THE BASICS OF VEGAN COOKING 25

CHAPTER 4: CREATING A COMPLETE MEAL 31

CHAPTER 5: SPECIAL NUTRITIONAL CONSIDERATIONS 37

APPETIZERS 41

Black Olive Hummus 43

Grilled Vegetable Skewers 44

BEVERAGES 45

Dr. Monique's Mango Muddled Mint Mock Mo-garita 47

Lemon, Ginger, and Basil Water 48

Homemade Orange Juice 48

BREADS 49

Vegan Cornbread 51

Vegan Zucchini Bread 52

BREAKFAST 53

Avocado Waffles 55

Chocolate Quinoa 56

Sweet Potato Hash 57

Handful Smoothie 58

DESSERTS 59

Mitchell's Vegan and Gluten-Free Chocolate Cake 61

Vegan and Gluten-Free Lemon Pound Cake with Lemon-Lime Glaze 63

Vegan and Gluten-Free Sweet Potato Pound Cake with Maple Orange Glaze.......65
Vegan Blondies.......67
ENTRÉES....... 69
Avocado Melt with Basil and Arugula Pesto.......71
Vegan Bean Tacos.......72
Quinoa and Mushroom Stuffed Peppers.......73
Spicy Vegan Potato Curry.......74
Philly Cheeze “Steak” Sandwich.......75
Jerk Tofu.......76
Pulled “Pork” with Homemade BBQ Sauce.......77
16-Bean Medley with Plant-Based Sausage and Purple Rice.......78
Cauliflower Rice Stir-Fry with Duck Sauce and Hot Mustard.......80
Vegan Lentil, Kale, and Sausage Pasta.......81
Red Rice, Brown Lentil, and Mushroom Burger.......82
Tofu Parmigiana.......83
Vegan “Butter Chicken”.......84
BBQ Ribz.......86
“Crab” Cakes.......88
Southwestern Bowl.......89
Vegan Lentil Tacos.......90
SALADS....... 91
Fresh Fruit Salad.......93
Mexican-Inspired Refrigerator “Clean Out”.......94
Super Salad.......95
Tricolor Pasta and Red Bean Salad.......96
Vegan Caesar Salad.......97
SAUCES AND GLAZES....... 99
Mexican Pesto....... 101
Raspberry Soy Sauce Glaze....... 102
Asian-Inspired Marinade....... 102
Mitchell and Mom’s Spaghetti Sauce....... 103

Dark Chocolate Balsamic Glaze 104
Vegan Alfredo Sauce 104
Vegan Green Goddess Dressing 105
Lime Cilantro Dressing 106

SIDE DISHES 107
Grandma's Fried Corn 109
Vegan Southern Baked Beans 110
Mommy's Cole Slaw 111
Cheezee Vegan Mac 'N' Cheeze 112
Cilantro Lime Rice 113

SOUPS 115
Vegan Black Bean Soup 117
Kale, Sausage, Red Potato, and Cannellini Bean Soup 118
Carrot Soup 119
Greek-Style Chickpea Soup 120
Classic Minestrone Soup 121

MY VEGAN-*ISH* JOURNEY 123

DR. MONIQUE'S FAVORITE VEGAN FOOD ABCs 125

APPENDIX 165

REFERENCES 169

ABOUT THE AUTHOR 171

Foreword

"Tribute to whom tribute is due, honor to whom honor."
—Romans 13:7

To our determined, dedicated, and delightful daughter, Dr. Monique May, board-certified family physician and "Physician in The Kitchen":

It is our pleasure to congratulate and applaud you as an author. Monique, you were heaven-sent to us and so many others. We recognized your uniqueness at a very young age. Your career choice and arduous undertaking to become a physician—and a *good* physician you are—speak to that. You have blessed so many lives. During all of your accomplishments (and there are many), you have been a loving, devoted, and wonderful mother to your son (our grandson) Mitchell. We are so happy for the affluent yet selfless lifestyle you have made for him as well as yourself.

Also, we are grateful that you have been inspired to share your wisdom, knowledge, and understanding of healthy living by writing this cookbook. Your care and concern for others will be demonstrated throughout this book, along with the delicious, healthy recipes and valuable information provided.

We thank the Lord for you, dear daughter!

The ancestors are joining us in our salutes, admiration, and overall accolades to our most deserving daughter, doctor, mother, mentor, and more.

Many will benefit from your labor.

Your loving parents,

Tedd and Hazel May

Introduction

What a wonderful—and delicious—journey this has been! When I decided to write a cookbook, all I knew was that I wanted to share my love for good food and healthy options with the world. Well, my own personal journey toward more plant-based meals happened along the way and has totally infused the direction of this book. And I could not be happier! Writing this book during the COVID-19 pandemic when eating the best foods that one has access to was even more vital was very timely for me personally. I was fortunate to turn 50 in May of 2020, and even though my celebration did not look like the one I thought I was going to have, I was still very grateful to have reached the half-century mark.

Reaching such a milestone certainly makes one reflect and pause to take stock of one's life, even more so against the backdrop of a global pandemic, to say the least. I asked myself the usual questions: How do I want the next five years, ten years, twenty-five years, even fifty years to look for me? What should I start doing now to improve my health and well-being? What activities should I stop? What things am I doing right, and should I continue to do them? And lastly, what changes can I make to ensure I step into my second half-century as fabulously as my first?

Well, to answer these questions, I bought a new house with a bigger, more spacious kitchen *(you know, to cook all this delicious food in!)*, joined the Peloton tribe, and most importantly, explored eating a more plant-based diet. At this stage of my journey, I describe myself as vegan-*ish,* meaning I still eat some animal products such as poultry, fish, and honey (I can't drink tea without it!); but by and large, the majority of what I eat is plant-based.

But this journey, which I began blogging about on my website (www.DrMoniqueMay.com), has been very exciting, challenging, educational, and rewarding! I have noticed improvements in my achy knees (yep, they're fifty-plus alright) and my blood pressure that I attribute to what I have been eating. In fact, the idea behind *Doc, Fix My Plate! The Physician in The Kitchen's Prescriptions for Your Healthy Meal Makeover* is a simple one. As a family medicine physician for more than twenty years, I spent my clinical career educating patients on ways to improve their health through lifestyle changes such as proper diet and exercise. As a social media influencer, I now use my platform to share my latest kitchen creations with my followers and educate them on the health benefits of food. This cookbook is a mash-up of those two passions. I am eager to try new plant-based substitutes and get an absolute thrill out of "vegan-izing" dishes like chicken and waffles, burgers, brownies, and even crab cakes! In this book, I will share these and other amazing recipes (or as I like to call them, prescriptions for healthy plate makeovers). I will also share my experiences, successes, failures, and *aha* moments.

In short, this book is a celebration! I am celebrating my new dietary discoveries, writing my second book, and most importantly, I am celebrating *life*! I am so looking forward to where this journey will lead, and so grateful that you have decided to come along for the ride!

See you in the kitchen,

Dr.Monique

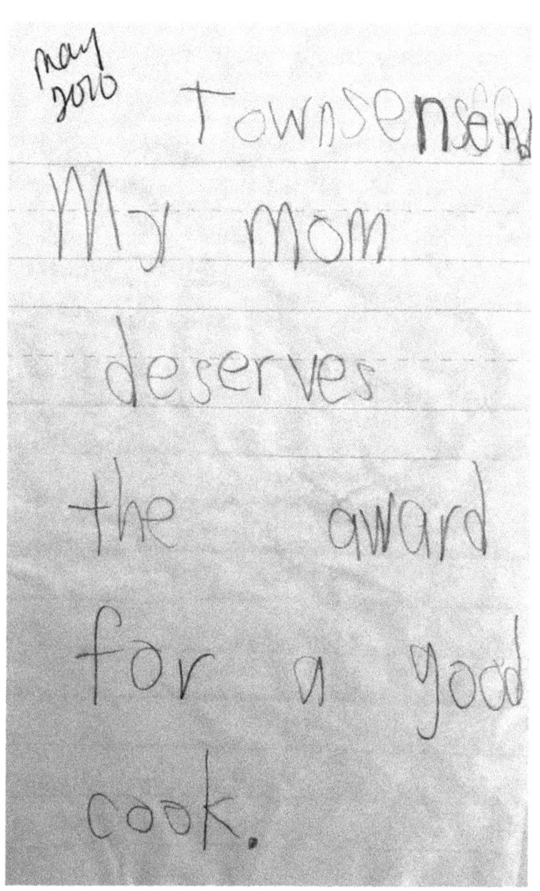

Unsolicited testimonal from my #1 fan, Mitchell, age 6.
That kid was onto something, huh? ☺

Chapter 1:
VEGAN BASICS 101

To make sure we are all on the same page, let's cover a few basics, shall we?

SO, WHAT DOES IT MEAN TO BE VEGAN, ANYWAY?

Veganism is a subset of vegetarianism. Some vegetarians still drink cow's or goat's milk and eat eggs, but not vegans. Vegans do not allow *any* animal products in their diet. They do not eat animal products or by-products of animal products, including seafood or fish. This means that they have to be creative in replacing commonly used foods such as eggs, milk, and meat. While the majority of the recipes in this book are vegan, since I consider myself to be vegan-*ish*, or more technically, flexitarian (meaning I eat mostly plants but also some poultry and fish), I have included some recipes that may be made with poultry as well.

VEGAN OR NAH?

In order for food to be vegan, it needs to meet certain criteria. It is important to note that there are a lot of hidden ingredients in foods, such as gelatin, lard (animal fat), and whey (the watery part of milk), which is why reading labels is very important. For example, I did not realize until recently that lemon curd contains eggs, so unfortunately, it is not vegan. Since bees are in the animal kingdom, vegans cannot eat honey, royal jelly, and bee pollen supplements. If you are a new vegan, making all of these changes may seem overwhelming and even expensive, but hopefully this book will help ease these concerns.

WHAT IS VEGAN COOKING?

Simply put, vegan cooking uses only non-animal sources to prepare meals. It is plant-based. It is flavorful, nutritious, and Physician in The Kitchen-approved!

Over the course of this book, we will peel back the (onion) layers of vegan cooking. This book will teach you many things, including the ABCs on how to cook vegan food correctly, typical ingredients used in vegan cooking, and how to stock a complete vegan pantry so you can prepare vegan dishes every day without a hassle. You will also learn how to put together a complete vegan meal containing the right balance of necessary vitamins, minerals, and nutrients. As a bonus, I will include my top choices for kitchen utensils, gadgets, and appliances.

TYPICAL INGREDIENTS IN VEGAN COOKING

Since vegan cooking is cooking is done without meat, fish, eggs, or any animal by-products, extra care needs to be taken to make sure that none of these ingredients are used. This section will focus on several different kinds of ingredients used in vegan cooking. First, we will learn how to replace milk and eggs with foods that are vegan-friendly. We will also cover other ingredients that are used in vegan cooking, as well as how to avoid animal by-products that may be hidden in processed foods.

REPLACING EGGS IN RECIPES

It can be a challenge to replace eggs in a recipe in order to make it vegan. Believe me, I know. Creating my line of vegan and gluten-free pound cakes was challenging for that very reason. Coming up with the right egg replacement took several efforts, but luckily for you, I have done the very hard work (and have included a few of those recipes in this book), and I learned quite a bit in the process. Because they are used so ubiquitously, eggs are one of the most difficult ingredients to replace. Fortunately, there are many options to choose from that will get the job done.

WHAT DO EGGS DO IN A RECIPE?

In most recipes, eggs are pretty much essential for the functions they serve, including:

- binding ingredients together
- making baked goods light and fluffy and helping them rise
- providing structure to the finished product
- providing extra moisture to baked goods

Eggs are especially useful in making baked goods and are essential for certain savory dishes (think quiche and frittatas) as well.

EGG REPLACEMENT OPTIONS

Here is a list of several vegan egg replacement options. You can replace the eggs in any recipe using these options. Keep your other ingredients and how you want your finished product to look, taste, and feel in mind. This will help you choose the correct substitute. To keep it simple, I have included the "egg math" for you for each option.

Aquafaba: Literally translated from the Latin "bean water," this is the liquid in any can of beans; but typically, chickpeas (garbanzo beans) or white navy beans are used due to their milder flavor. This magical liquid that I admittedly had been pouring down the drain for years can fill the role of egg whites in meringues and mousses. It can act as a binder, leavening agent, or emulsifier. You will not believe how my moist and addictive **Vegan Blondies** are made from an entire can of navy beans (beans plus the juice) until you try it for yourself. I was super excited to discover this much healthier alternative to eggs and have used it in a variety of ways, with my friends and family none the wiser.

Pureed Bananas: Pureed bananas are a creamy and effective egg substitute. Place a ripe banana in your blender and puree until completely smooth. One half of a regular-sized banana equals one egg. Bananas are readily available and very economical. However, bananas have a distinct taste that does not work well in every recipe. For example, if you are making peanut butter cookies, adding banana would not work in your f(l)avor (unless you are making them Elvis Presley-style).

Ground Flaxseeds: Flax is a plant with many health benefits, including reducing the risk for heart disease, cancer, stroke, and diabetes. It contains the "good fat" omega-3 fatty acids, which are good for your heart. Flax also contains fiber and antioxidant properties due to lignans, which are beneficial plant chemicals. Flaxseeds are used in a lot of foods, such as whole-grain breads, cereals, and snacks. When using them at home, it is ideal to purchase the flaxseeds whole and store them in the refrigerator. Process them in a blender or coffee grinder. However, for the sake of time and convenience, I purchase ground flaxseeds and skip this step. To make your "flegg" for each egg called for in a recipe. Use 1 tablespoon of flaxseeds for every egg that you need to replace and add 2–3 tablespoons of water to each tablespoon of ground flaxseeds. Add the water slowly while whisking vigorously. Whisk until the mixture takes on a gel-like consistency. Let sit for at least 10 minutes. Refrigerating the mixture helps to speed up the process. Since flaxseeds have a nutty taste, use this egg replacement for making things like whole-grain breads, muffins, and pancakes. Experiment with your recipes so you can get an idea of the types of items in which you would use this option.

Chia Seeds: Chia seeds are the edible seeds of the chia plant. They too are rich in fiber, omega-3 fatty acids, and antioxidants, as well as iron and calcium. Just like with ground flaxseeds, the math is super easy here, too: 1 tablespoon of chia seeds plus 3 tablespoons of water equals 1 chia egg (a "chegg" dare I say?). Again, let the mixture set for 10 minutes, refrigerating if desired. However, due to their dark color (unless you use white chia seeds), I would recommend using chia seeds only in darker items like chocolate cake, brownies, or zucchini bread.

Ripe Avocadoes: As an avowed avocadoholic, I never need an excuse to include an avocado in a dish. But how much more awesome is it to know that these beauties can also be the egg's much healthier and prettier understudy and can even steal the show? What a coincidence that avocadoes are shaped like eggs, too! Anywho, I used ripe avocadoes instead of eggs to create my vegan **Avocado Waffles** that I have included in this book for you to try. The pretty flecks of green they add to the batter are an additional bonus. Just think of what a kitchen rock star your family will think you are when you serve them green-tinged waffles for St. Patrick's Day next year! Be warned: once you go avocado, you may never go back. For the avocado newbie, fret not: avocadoes have a mild-enough taste that they do not alter your plans for your dish. For more on the health benefits of avocadoes, see A is for Avocado on Dr. Monique's Favorite Vegan Foods ABCs list at the end of this book.

Tofu: Tofu is another egg replacement option you can try. Tofu is made from soybeans and water. It is then pressed into blocks and comes in different textures: silken, medium, and firm or extra firm. For a scrambled egg replacement, I use the firm texture and add turmeric to give it that classic yellow color. To replace binding ingredients and thickening agents in baked goods, silken tofu seems to yield the best results.

The nice thing about tofu is that it blends well with most flavors. Flaxseeds, in contrast, have a distinct nutty flavor. Tofu is very bland on its own and pairs well with stronger ingredients. Another benefit is that it is widely available in most areas, even in regular supermarkets. To use, just blend or puree the tofu until it is smooth in your blender. A food processor also may work, but it is important to make sure that there are no lumps and that the texture is as smooth as possible. To replace 1 large egg, use ¼ cup of the pureed mixture for each egg. The same amount of unflavored soy yogurt will work just as well.

You will likely need to do some experimenting to see which recipes work best with tofu as an egg substitute. As is the case with all of these substitutes, it all depends on the kinds of recipes you try and your personal preferences.

Commercial Egg Replacement Products: There are several vegan-friendly egg replacement products available at your local store. Read the packaging to make sure they are truly vegan and that they do not contain any animal by-products. They come in both powder and refrigerated liquid forms.

Egg replacement powders get mixed reviews. Some people like them a lot, others not so much. They are definitely convenient and good to have on hand. Once you get used to cooking vegan, you will start to learn your preferences and identify your must-haves.

Since there are several brands on the market, it may take a while to find one that you like the most. When using these items, be sure to follow the package instructions. Be on the lookout for them in your local grocery store, health food store, or online.

Honorable egg replacement mentions include **applesauce, black salt, tapioca starch,** and **chickpea flour**. A simple Google search will show you many recipes that feature these egg replacement options. Go forth and experiment!

Using Flour and Other Leavening Agents

Leavening agents lighten and aerate batters. Also known as raising agents, they help cakes and other baked goods rise while baking by adding carbon dioxide (yes, baking is really just a big old, delicious chemistry experiment).

You can also use pastes made from different kinds of flours and leavening agents to replace eggs. The bonus is that most people already have these ingredients on hand. These pastes also do not have flavors of their own like bananas and flaxseeds do. They can blend into batters fairly easily. However, you may have to experiment to get the proportions just right. Here are some suggestions (by the way, baking is also a bit of math as well):

- 1 tablespoon flour of any kind, such as wheat, oat, or soy flour + 1 tablespoon water = 1 egg. If using gluten-free flour, you may need to add xanthan gum for structure and moisture. Verify what your particular gluten-free flour calls for and follow the directions to create the outcome you desire.
- 1 tablespoon baking powder + 1 tablespoon flour + 2 tablespoons water blended together = 1 egg.
- 2 tablespoons corn starch + 2 tablespoons water blended together = 1 egg.

FINDING THE RIGHT EGG SUBSTITUTE

I lovingly refer to my kitchen as my "lab" because as simple as cooking can be, there is some trial and error, especially when it comes to baking. Keeping track of what works and does not work will save time, ingredients, and stress, to say the least. As you try these different combinations, you will get a feel for which egg substitutes work best for which recipes. Try making one of your favorite dishes using different egg substitutes until you achieve the flavor and texture you desire.

For example, if you want to make blueberry muffins, try any one of these substitutions in place of eggs. Then make a note of how it tastes. Next time you make it, try a different egg substitute. Each time you try one, jot down notes about texture, moisture, taste, crumb, etc. After trying several options, think about which one was your favorite and stick with that. Pretty soon, you will be able to tell fairly easily which egg replacement products work best for certain kinds of recipes. I keep a simple notebook handy in the lab as I am creating new recipes for this very reason.

REPLACING MILK IN RECIPES

For a vegan, milk from any animal (sheep, cow, goat) is not an option. However, milk is a common ingredient in baking and cooking. Fortunately, it is much easier to replace than eggs. To replace milk in recipes, just substitute any of these vegan alternatives. For example, if the recipe calls for 1 cup of milk, use 1 cup of soy milk instead. Here are some alternative milk options:

Soy Milk: Soy milk comes in a variety of flavors and is readily available. Flavors include vanilla, unsweetened, chocolate, and even eggnog. Some brands are thicker and creamier than others. Experiment to find the brands you like the best. Regular soy milk is fairly neutral and blends well in recipes. It is also rich in protein.

Nut Milks: Nut milks include almond milk and hazelnut milk. Unlike soy milk, these nut milks have their own distinct flavors and may clash with certain recipes. That being said, I use almond milk pretty much exclusively without perceiving any effect on the taste. There are sweetened and unsweetened varieties as well. People who are allergic to nuts should avoid this group.

Rice Milk: Rice milk is another option for milk replacement. It is very mild-tasting and blends well in recipes. However, it is important to note that rice milk typically does not contain a lot of protein (compared to soy and nut milks). That just means you would need to get more protein from other sources. Rest assured, as you become familiar with the different flavors of these plant milks, you will get a feel for the recipes in which they work best.

REPLACING BUTTERMILK IN RECIPES

Buttermilk is also an important ingredient used in several different recipes. It adds tanginess, moisture, and acidity to cakes, biscuits, and cornbread. Just as importantly, it contributes to the "crumb" of the good pound cake that we know and love. For vegans, using regular buttermilk is not an option. But buttermilk is just milk that has been to the opera: in other words, it is "cultured." It contains some good bacteria in it just like yogurt does. Even better, it is super easy to make your own. This recipe makes 1 cup of vegan-friendly "buttermilk":

1. Measure 1 cup of plant milk in a glass measuring cup.
2. Add 1 tablespoon of acid (vinegar or lemon juice) and mix well.
3. Let the mixture sit for about 5–15 minutes before using it.

Soy milk works the best. Rice milk and nut milks do not work as well (again, chemistry).

REPLACING BUTTER OR FAT IN RECIPES

Butter and some forms of fat are important ingredients used in a lot of recipes. There are several ways to substitute them:

Plant Butter: This is my go-to for baking and cooking, but like regular butter, it must be used in moderation. Sold under a variety of brand names, plant butter is usually a blend of plant-based oils such as avocado, olive, and almond oil. It may also contain palm kernel or coconut oil and other additives such as salt, colorings, and natural or artificial flavors to give them the taste and feel of regular butter. They may also contain more omega-6 fatty acids, which have been linked to inflammation. Compared to animal butter, plant butters are cholesterol-free and tend to have less saturated fat (unhealthy fat) and more mono- and polyunsaturated fat (healthier fat). Plant butters may be slightly higher in sodium than animal butters. When using these, look for ones that are not as processed and contain no artificial additives. Be aware that palm and coconut oils contain high levels of saturated fat, so be mindful of that. Environmentally, palm oil is a bit controversial due to the way it is harvested. Hopefully, this will improve with time.

Vegetable Oil: If the recipe calls for melted or even solid butter, you can use vegetable oil instead. This, however, may alter the texture of the recipe somewhat, so you will probably need to experiment. Out of all the available types of cooking oil, vegetable oil takes the prize for containing the highest levels of polyunsaturated fat, which we know decreases the risk for blocked arteries that lead to heart attacks. Extra-light olive oil has a mild taste and can be used in baking as well.

Coconut Oil: This oil has a high level of saturated fat (up to 82 percent, according to the American Heart Association, way more than the 10–20 percent that the other commonly used oils contain).[1] Coconut oil has been shown to raise the levels of low-density lipoproteins (LDL cholesterol, the bad cholesterol), similar to the effects of butter. It also raises LDL more than olive oil. For vegans, coconut oil may provide the saturated fats they may not otherwise get. For meat-eaters, however, it is not recommended. Saturated fats should comprise no more than 7 to 10 percent of your total calories per day. For a 2,000-calorie diet, that is 140–200 calories or 16–22 grams of saturated fat per day.

Fruit Purees: Fruit purees can be used to reduce the fat in recipes that call for butter. For example, if the recipe calls for 1 cup of butter, use ½ cup apple sauce and ½ cup vegan margarine or butter. Other fruit purees include plum puree and banana puree. Just make sure they are vegan-friendly and low in sugar. Depending on what you are making, you may also want to try replacing all the fat in the recipe with fruit. This may work well with tarts, pies, or cakes.

Shortening and Margarine: I mention these here only to recommend that you *avoid* them, as they are highly processed and contain artificial trans fats. These fats, which are a subtype of unsaturated fat, are the result of the chemical processing of vegetable oils to give them a longer shelf-life in products such as cakes, muffins, doughnuts, potato chips, microwave popcorn, and fried fast foods such as chicken, hamburgers, and french fries. Read your labels carefully and do not buy anything that has "partially hydrogenated oil" in the ingredient list.

At the end of the day, always make sure that butter and fat replacement products are used in moderation. A diet that is high in fat and trans fats is not a healthy diet. If you absolutely need them, use the least amount that you can.

COMMON INGREDIENTS USED IN VEGAN COOKING

As demonstrated in the previous section, ingredients such as milk, buttermilk, eggs, and butter are almost essential for certain recipes. But as we have seen, the substitutions are more than adequate and healthier for you. With that said, there are several more ingredients that many vegan chefs find essential.

Here is a rundown of some commonly used soy items:

SOY PRODUCTS

Soy is a very versatile product, especially when it comes to creating healthy, protein-rich vegan meals. Here is a list of some soy products that are available, a few of which we have already touched upon:

- **Soy milk:** Easy-to-find and comes in several different flavors such as vanilla and chocolate. It can be sweetened or unsweetened.
- **Tofu:** As mentioned previously, tofu comes in different levels of firmness such as extra-firm or soft. It is rich in calcium and iron.
- **Tempeh:** Tempeh is a fermented product with a hearty, meaty texture that can be used in stir-fries, burgers, tacos, sandwiches, and even in place of bacon. It is rich in protein.
- **Ground meat replacement:** This soy product can be used to make meatballs, tacos, and vegan chili. Use products with ingredients that are easy to pronounce and not highly processed.
- **Soy yogurt:** Soy yogurt contains active cultures just like regular yogurt and comes in a variety of flavors.
- **Miso:** Miso is a fermented, salty paste that is made from soy and is popular as an enzyme-rich soup base or marinade. It is used to add umami flavor to vegan dishes.
- **Tamari and soy sauce:** Both condiments are made from soy and are used in Asian cooking. Tamari, however, is gluten-free. It contains less sodium than soy sauce.
- **Edamame**: These soybeans are excellent by themselves as a healthy snack or in stir-fries.
- **Soy cheese:** Soy cheese melts and has a texture similar to dairy cheese.
- **Soy sausage, hot dogs, and hamburger patties:** Vegans can enjoy breakfast sausage, hot dogs, and even hamburger patties made from soy. However, avoid highly processed products with more chemicals than ingredients you can pronounce.
- **Soy "chicken":** Another meat replacement option, it comes in a variety of forms such as patties, nuggets, etc. Same precautions as mentioned above.

- **Soy protein powder:** Soy protein offers a great way to increase your daily protein intake. You can put a scoop in your morning smoothie or add it to recipes such as pancakes and quick breads.
- **Soy flour:** This is a gluten-free option for baking that people who avoid gluten can use.

There are a variety of soy products available, and this is just a partial list. It simply illustrates how versatile soy is. Look for soy products that are made from non-genetically modified soybeans.

Interestingly, soy foods do have their critics. Purists may only like to use them in their "traditional" forms such as tofu, tempeh, miso, edamame, and tamari. Opponents of processed soy products are leery of the fact that they are designed to taste like meat or milk products, which to them defeats the purpose of being vegan. Also, these foods tend to be highly processed, which does not make them healthier. Whether or not you decide to use them is a decision that you should make after you weigh the pros and cons. Remember, just because something is labeled "natural," "vegan," or even "organic" does not mean it is necessarily good for you. You still must be an educated consumer and read your labels so you can make the best food choices possible. For example, some soy hot dogs and burgers are highly processed and contain high amounts of sodium and fat.

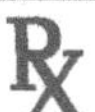 **DOCTOR'S NOTES**

One other "controversy" around soy: Some breast cancer survivors avoid eating soy due to concerns that it may increase the chance that their breast cancer may return. Soy contains phytoestrogens, which actually work on the same receptors as your natural estrogen but instead block their effects. Interestingly, studies in women with breast cancer have actually shown a protective effect of eating soy and a decreased risk of breast cancer recurrence and higher survival rates.[2] This may explain, in part, why women in Asia who eat a lot of soy have lower breast cancer rates than we have in the United States. They also tend to have much milder menopause symptoms.

WHOLE GRAINS

So many grains, so little time! There are so many different kinds of whole grains out there; it is worthwhile to take the time and experiment. Grains are rich in carbohydrates, vitamins, minerals, fiber, and other important nutrients. They even have protein, especially quinoa—an ancient grain that is especially protein-rich.

Here are some whole grains to add to your repertoire:

- Rye
- Buckwheat
- Quinoa (a complete protein because it contains all 9 essential amino acids that we cannot make ourselves)
- Oats
- Brown rice
- Ancient grains such as farro, amaranth, barley, bulgur, wheat berries, and millet

These can be ground into flour or eaten whole. They should form the backbone of a healthy vegan diet. Whole wheat products (for example, pasta) and popcorn (yes, you read that correctly!) are options as well. But just like anything else that starts off healthy, popcorn can be sabotaged by what you add to it, so make good choices.

NUTS AND SEEDS

Nuts and seeds are another essential (and delicious) part of a healthy vegan diet. They are rich in vitamins, minerals, and important nutrients like proteins, carbohydrates, and healthy fats.

Here is a list of some nuts and seeds to consider adding to your diet:

- Hazelnuts
- Walnuts
- Sunflower seeds
- Pumpkin seeds
- Pecans
- Almonds
- Cashews
- Sesame seeds
- Poppy seeds
- Flaxseeds
- Hemp seeds

Use them in recipes (salad toppings, for example) or eat them by themselves as a snack. Roasting them in the oven or toasting them on the stovetop takes their flavors up a notch. Add ground flaxseeds or chia seeds to your morning smoothies. And yes, nut butters count too!

LEGUMES

Legumes are an essential protein source for vegans, especially when paired with whole grains. They can be combined to create meals with complete nutrient profiles. If legumes are one of your main protein sources, remember to combine them with other plant-based options.

Here are just a few examples. This list is by no means exhaustive:

- Chickpeas (garbanzo beans)
- Lentils
- Kidney beans
- Black beans
- Cannellini beans
- Northern beans
- Black-eyed peas
- Split peas
- Soybeans
- Peanuts (These are different from the nuts listed above because they grow in underground pods instead of on trees.)

Legumes come in dried form, ground into flour, or canned. The dried form needs to be soaked overnight to soften them or—my personal favorite way—cooked in a pressure cooker. The canned variety is easy to use and great to have on hand. Remember that aquafaba I talked about earlier? Well, this is where it comes from. Legume flours are becoming increasingly popular ingredients in baked foods and savory cooking. They offer a gluten-free option for those who prefer not to use wheat flour.

FRUITS AND VEGETABLES

Vital for good health, fruits and vegetables add color and variety to your meals (#eatyourcolors). Aim for 5–12 servings per day to get all the vitamins, minerals, and nutrients that you need daily. Believe it or not, the average healthy adult really does not need to take vitamin supplements if he or she just follows this simple rule, vegan or not.

Use organic produce whenever possible and affordable. Organically grown produce is grown without using chemical pesticides or fertilizers. Organic food is also better for the environment. However, if you want to save money, you don't have to buy everything organic. Peaches, strawberries, nectarines, sweet potatoes, carrots, green beans, and sweet bell peppers are just a few items that are recommended to buy organic. Conventionally grown grapes, apples, bananas, blueberries, tomatoes, broccoli, and onions are okay to buy, depending on where they are from (i.e., country of origin; produce grown in the US is not always the best due to contamination from pesticides). Buying seasonal, local produce is ideal, as it helps support your local economy and it often tastes a lot fresher. Don't forget to stock your freezer with frozen fruits and veggies to enjoy year-round.

CANNED AND PACKAGED FOODS

As the vegan diet increases in popularity, so does the availability of packaged, vegan foods. Below is a list of some available items:

- Breads
- Desserts
- Baked goods
- Snacks
- Vegan chocolate
- Canned goods
- Beverages
- Breakfast foods and cereals

Again, just because something is labeled as vegan does not mean that you don't have to read the labels or look for additives, chemicals, and processed fillers.

HOW TO SPOT HIDDEN NON-VEGAN INGREDIENTS

As mentioned before, there are often hidden ingredients in foods that are animal byproducts. An educated vegan will take the extra step needed to investigate what these ingredients are and avoid them.

If a packaged food is listed as vegan-friendly, you can be fairly confident that it does not contain hidden non-vegan ingredients in it. But it is still a good idea to check. Below is a list of ingredients to avoid. There are two types of ingredients—those that are clearly from animal products and those that may be from either animal *or* plant products.

If the ingredient falls in the second category, you may need to do a little research on the food product to find out if it is derived from a plant or an animal. That can take some effort, so when in doubt, just leave it out.

HIDDEN ANIMAL-DERIVED INGREDIENTS

When I say hidden ingredients, I simply mean that it may not be obvious that these ingredients are actually animal-derived. These ingredients are often used in foods, and vegan products should not contain these. Check the ingredients list to make sure these are not included:

- Albumin – a protein that comes from egg whites
- Milk products – including whey protein powder, lactase, lactose, and of course, milk and dried milk
- Calcium caseinate – a commonly used additive used to increase the protein and calcium content of processed foods. It works as an emulsifier, thickener, and stabilizer.
- Calcium stearate – another additive used in spices, dry mixes, dietary supplements, and prescription medicines. An anti-caking agent, it works as a binder and lubricant.
- Suet – a type of animal fat
- Tallow – an animal fat product made from suet used to make candles and soap
- Bee products – including royal jelly, propolis, honey, and bee pollen
- Carmine – a food additive that comes from insects
- Lard – a type of animal fat
- Casein – the protein found in cheese
- Gelatin – a popular product frequently found in jellies and desserts; commonly derived from animal collagen

Other common hidden ingredients derived from animals include:

- Cochineal
- Isinglass

- Muriatic acid
- Oleic acid
- Palmitic acid
- Pancreatin
- Pepsin

Most of the above ingredients are typically used as additives in foods. They have different purposes, depending on the food in which they are used.

INGREDIENTS THAT MAY BE FROM ANIMALS

The following ingredients serve different functions in food. Some are considered additives. Others emulsify foods and supply extra fats. However, just because an ingredient sounds like an animal ingredient does not mean it is. It could be synthetically manufactured or derived from plants. You will need to check.

These ingredients are:

- Emulsifying agents
- Fatty acid
- Adipic acid
- Glyceride
- Glycerol
- Capric acid
- Lactic acid
- Magnesium stearate
- Monoglyceride
- Anything listed as "natural flavoring"
- Clarifying agents
- Disodium inosinate
- Glyceride
- Glycerol
- Stearic acid

- Diglyceride
- Polysorbate
- Sodium stearoyl lactylate (a source of salt as well)

Yes, some of these ingredients are hard to say—some of them sound like something you learned in chemistry class! They all have different purposes in the foods that we eat on a daily basis, even foods that we may not think to consider. The point is that if you truly want to follow a vegan diet, it is worth the extra step to determine if your favorite foods use the animal-derived versions of these ingredients. Or better yet, if any of these items are one of the first five ingredients listed on the package, just put it back (ingredients are listed in descending order, so the first item is present in the highest quantity). Better still, if they appear *anywhere* in the ingredient list, avoid the food product altogether. It is best not to eat things you cannot pronounce. Think about it: when you write your grocery list, are you writing down *stearic acid* or *sodium stearoyl lactylate*? I highly doubt it.

Vegan or not, the fewer processed foods you eat, the better. That is why produce is truly the perfect whole food—it comes in its own packaging, and other than possible pesticides (and the occasional bacterial contamination), you never have to worry about what is in it. It is important to realize that the ingredients mentioned in this section can be found in almost everything. However, if you focus on analyzing food labels too much, it may get overwhelming and paralyzing. Keep things simple and stress-free, especially if you are just starting on your vegan journey. If you are new to reading package labels, start by making sure that the first five to ten ingredients listed (hopefully, there are no more than that) are easy to read and pronounce. Over time, you will become more adept at knowing what is good for you to eat and what is not. Do what you need to do in order to make informed decisions so you can eat as healthy as you can.

Being a vegan is definitely a lifestyle commitment. Learning about the foods you need to eat, making vegan-friendly substitutions while baking and cooking, and educating yourself about the ingredients you may want to avoid are all necessary parts of embracing the vegan lifestyle. Hopefully, this chapter will help start you off on the right track.

Chapter 2:

SETTING UP THE VEGAN PANTRY

Now that we have learned what to eat and look for in our food labels, let's use that information to stock and organize our vegan kitchen pantry. Setting up your pantry is an essential step to being able to meal plan for the week or easily create meals on a whim. If you have been vegan or vegetarian all of your life, setting up your pantry should be fairly easy. However, if you have just recently committed to going vegan, you will probably need to start from scratch. You may have some basic ingredients on hand, but most of your pantry may not be vegan-friendly. Keep in mind that when I say "pantry," I am also referring to your freezer and cabinets or wherever you store your food. You should always "shop" from your pantry first and then buy what you need as you go. This saves money and time, as well as food. Remember that dried and frozen foods have "best used by" dates, and you do not want to lose good, nutritious food to spoilage or freezer burn.

Of course, you would not store perishable items such as fruits and vegetables in your pantry. However, some items, such as plant milks and certain brands of tofu, can be stored on the shelves and not in the refrigerator due to their packaging. Once they are opened, of course, they must be refrigerated.

STEP ONE: TAKE INVENTORY

The first step of building a vegan pantry is to take inventory of what you have. This step is mostly for those who have just become vegan. However, even if you have been vegan for a while, you will also benefit from this. The goal is to go through your food and think about everything you have and determine if it supports the vegan lifestyle or what your tastes and needs are now.

You may also want to look at the ingredient lists on all of your packaged foods to see if any of the hidden ingredients listed in the previous chapter are lurking. Even if you have been vegan for a while, you may still find some foods in your pantry that should not be there.

If you do find some food you want to get rid of and it has not been opened yet, do not throw it away. Give it to a local food pantry. Just because you will not eat it does not mean that someone else will not benefit from it. They may appreciate having something to eat. Be a blessing to someone else.

STEP TWO: STOCK THE ESSENTIALS

It is not entirely necessary to have a large pantry filled with tons of ingredients and packaged foods. Just think about the types of foods that are really important to you. If you do not bake too often, for example, do not bother buying baking supplies until you really need them. If you are the type of person who loves cereal and has a few bowls per day, you may want to keep a variety of plant milks and extra cereal in your pantry so you do not need to run to the store all the time.

Once you figure out what you need and what your eating preferences are, then you can start stocking your pantry. If you do not take the extra time to think about what you need, you may purchase things you will not eat and then the food will go to waste. Just stock the essentials, and if you need other things, you can buy them as you go along.

STEP THREE: ONLY PURCHASE WHAT YOU NEED

It can be expensive to stock your pantry all at once. There are certain ingredients that you may need once in a while, such as special kinds of beans or other items. It is not crucial to buy these extras at first. You can add to your pantry gradually as you go shopping or as the need arises.

In general, it is nice to have the ingredients on hand to make a few simple meals such as pasta dishes, soups, and grain and legume dinners such as rice and beans. Think about the kinds of foods you like to eat and keep a variety of those ingredients on hand.

If you are on a tight budget, consider buying some items in bulk, especially the ones you use often, such as almond milk, canned tomatoes, beans, or pasta. Look for sales at your local grocery store or warehouse clubs, and clip those digital coupons. Plan your meals in advance and write out a shopping list. Use foods that can be used in multiple dishes to keep the menu fresh. I talk more about this in my best-selling book, *MealMasters: Your Simple Guide to Modern-Day Meal Planning*. You can buy any special or extra items at the beginning of the week and use them as you need them.

EXAMPLE OF A VEGAN PANTRY

Even though pantries differ from household to household, it is helpful to review a sample pantry. Use this as a starting point when trying to figure out how to stock your kitchen, or you can take this list to the store and start shopping! Just have fun with it and make it your own!

It may help to think of your pantry in terms of categories. For example, my pantry is organized by breakfast items, baking goods, pasta and rice, milks, flavored water, etc.

Here is a sample list to get you started:

Breakfast Items

- Whole grain hot cereals such as oatmeal or quinoa
- Cold cereals, as well as plant milks
- Vegan pancake mixes
- Vegan baked goods (without the additives discussed in Chapter 1)

Snacks

- A variety of healthy snack items such as granola or protein bars
- Rice cakes
- Dried fruits, fruit roll-ups, fruit cups (avoid added sugars or syrups)
- Veggie chips
- Air-popped chips

Miscellaneous Items

- Nut milk, soy milk, oat milk, and rice milk (these are sold in special packaging that makes them pantry-friendly to stay fresh longer)
- Silken tofu (may be sold in packages that do not require refrigeration, unlike the medium and firm tofu you find in the refrigerated case in the produce aisle)
- Nuts and seeds such as almonds, sesame seeds, sunflower seeds, and pecans (remember, nut butters count as well)
- Capers (add a salty, briny, umami flavor to dishes; they are great for using in place of anchovies or sardines)
- Tomato products: spaghetti sauce, tomato sauce, marinara sauce, canned tomatoes (crushed, diced, whole, pureed), and tomato paste
- Canned jackfruit (can be used in place of pulled pork, chicken, or crab meat)
- Canned vegetables such as beans, artichokes, hearts of palm, etc. Look for low-sodium variations and rinse before using them. But save that aquafaba! (see Chapter 1)

Grain Products

- Brown, red, or purple rice
- Buckwheat flour
- Whole wheat flour
- Quinoa
- Whole wheat pasta
- Oatmeal
- Popcorn
- Barley
- Buckwheat

Condiments

- Vegetable oil
- At least one kind of flavorful oil, such as extra virgin olive oil or roasted sesame oil
- At least one oil with a high smoke point, such as avocado or peanut oil, for cooking at high heat
- Tamari and/or soy sauce
- Coconut aminos (a low-sodium, soy, and gluten-free option that adds savory flavor to meals and can be used in place of soy sauce. Despite the name, it does not taste like coconut.)
- Vinegar (keep several kinds on hand, such as apple cider, balsamic, rice wine, and red wine vinegar for a variety of flavors. Acid is very important in balancing seasoning and taste)
- Salt, pepper, herbs, and spices
- Organic ketchup
- Vegan mayonnaise (you can also make your own)
- Nutritional yeast (not the same as the yeast used for baking, used to make vegan cheeses and sauces)

Baking Items

- Leavening agents such as yeast, baking powder, and baking soda
- Vegan egg substitutes (see Chapter 1)
- A variety of flours
- Sugars and other sweetener products such as maple syrup

This list is meant only to be a starting point. It is impossible to come up with a complete list. Over time, it can be a matter of trial and error. Purchase new items one at a time and give them a try. You just may end up discovering something you will become obsessed with (quinoa, I'm looking at you)!

If you choose to stock your pantry with vegan packaged foods, remember to look at the ingredients. As previously mentioned, there are often hidden ingredients that are not vegan-friendly, not to mention unhealthy additives. When in doubt, leave it out—or better yet, make it yourself!

Chapter 3

THE BASICS OF VEGAN COOKING

Pop quiz: What have we covered so far? Well, since this is an open-book quiz—an open-cookbook quiz, that is—I will remind you.

In Chapter 1, we reviewed the basics of what it means to be vegan and talked about good replacements for egg, milk, and butter. In Chapter 2, we stocked our vegan pantry with all sorts of nonperishable goodies. Now it's time to start rattling some pots and pans and whip up some delicious magic in your kitchen! If you already know how to cook, awesome sauce; maybe you can skip this chapter. However, I do recommend reading it anyway because there may be tips and tricks in here you do not already know.

Learning how to cook, or learning new cooking techniques, can happen quickly or may evolve over time. It really depends on the person, their motivation to try new things, and their comfort level in the kitchen. Let's take a closer look at each step in the process. If you want to learn more, consider enrolling in a class (like my series on www.cookingwithDrMonique.com).

SETTING UP YOUR KITCHEN

As mentioned in the previous chapter, stocking your pantry is an important piece of the vegan-cooking puzzle. Having a well-equipped kitchen is nice, too. But don't fret if you just have the basics. As long as you can make delicious and satisfying meals with what you have, that is what counts! I am convinced that there are two types of cooks out there: those who like to use a lot of gadgets, and those who do not. I, dear reader, happen to fall in the first group (#kitchengadgetjunkie). Most home cooks likely fall somewhere in between.

Below is a list of some of the basic kitchen supplies you need to have on hand to be able to cook a variety of recipes:

- A good set of knives, including a bread knife and a chef's knife. Unless your knives are serrated, sharpen them regularly. Dull knives can be more dangerous than sharp ones. You will know it is time to sharpen them when you notice that cutting something is not as easy as it used to be. You will also want a large cutting board with grooves to catch liquids.

- An electric mixer. If you do a lot of baking, you may want to get a stand mixer that sits on your countertop; it frees up your hands so you can add ingredients quickly and do other things while it mixes your batter.
- Various cooking utensils, such as a pair of sturdy tongs, a colander, wooden spoons, rubber spatulas, and a wire whisk
- Small toaster oven
- Microwave oven
- Air fryer
- Blender and/or food processor
- Optional, but nice to have on hand: an immersion blender (also called a handheld blender), Crock-Pot or slow cooker, MultiPot or pressure cooker, ice cream maker, bread maker, vacuum sealer
- A variety of pots, pans, baking dishes, and mixing bowls

This list is not all-inclusive. If you come across a recipe that calls for specialized equipment, you can either buy it or make a substitution to save money. There is no need to go buy everything at once. The more you cook, the more you will start to understand your personal style and needs. For a list of my personal favorite gadgets and appliances, go to kit.co/DrMonique. For a more extensive list, see the Appendix.

FOLLOWING AND CREATING RECIPES

Learning how to follow recipes can be very helpful if you are starting to learn how to cook. Use recipes that are pretty straightforward. If you are new to cooking, you will likely be following recipes all the time. However, as you get more comfortable in the kitchen, you will gradually start to lose your dependence on them. After you follow a few recipes, you can start to write your own original creations down. Just remember to list the ingredients in the order that they will appear in the instructions. This makes the recipe easier to follow. Also, write down any substitutions or tips that were helpful to you while making your dish. Include how many servings you got out of the recipe as well. Keep in mind that recipes are really just guidelines or roadmaps; to paraphrase one of my favorite Peloton instructors, Denis: Recipes are suggestions, but you make the decisions to make a dish your own. This is especially true for savory dishes. When it comes to baking, I recommend following the recipe outright, at least the first time you try the recipe. Baking is more specific, like chemistry, and one wrong substitution or measurement can translate into disaster.

BASIC COOKING TECHNIQUES

After you set up your kitchen and make sure you understand how to follow recipes, the next step is to learn some basic cooking techniques. Here is a short list of some of the processes you will need to learn so you can cook.

LEARN HOW TO USE YOUR KNIVES

I may be showing my age here, but I swear I heard Keith Sweat singing when I wrote this next sentence: There is a right and wrong way to chop. (If you don't know who Keith Sweat is, Google him). Before now, you may not have given your chopping technique much thought. I know I didn't until I actually took a knife-skills cooking class. Talk about mind-blowing! However, the wrong technique can get you injured, make you inefficient, and affect how evenly your food is cooked. Always make sure your knives are sharp, too. As mentioned, knives can actually be more dangerous if they are dull. When a knife is dull, it does not cut well, and when you apply more pressure or saw back and forth to get it to cut, it can slip and cut you instead. Use the "claw" method: with the knife in your dominant hand, stabilize what you are cutting by gripping it with your index, middle, ring, and pinky fingers, with the thumb tucked just behind them. Using a rocking motion, move the knife through the item as you cut toward your other hand. By placing and tucking your fingers this way, you avoid cutting yourself and it helps make your cuts more even. As you get better, you can experiment with different types of cuts, such as the slice, julienne (produces matchstick-sized pieces), dice, mince, chop, cube, and chiffonade, to name a few. Keep in mind that the more consistent your pieces are, the more consistently they will cook. This makes a big difference in your cooking time and the consistency, taste, and appearance of your finished dish.

LEARN THE DIFFERENCE BETWEEN BOILING, HEATING, AND SIMMERING

These are three very basic cooking techniques for the stovetop:

- Boiling is when you set the heat on high and the liquid makes large bubbles, like when you boil eggs.
- Heating is when you let the food get hot but not boiling (so there won't be any bubbles). This is done over low-to-medium heat.

- Simmering is when you cook on low heat for a long amount of time, and there may be small, fine bubbles at the edges or on the surface. Dishes like soups and stews, for example, are typically simmered (think low and slow).

LEARN THE DIFFERENCE BETWEEN BAKING AND BROILING

The terms *baking* and *broiling* are not the same things. Both use the dry heat of an oven, but with baking, the food usually starts as liquid or mixture, and in broiling, it is typically a solid item. Some foods that can be baked can also be broiled and vice versa. Baking, however, occurs at a lower heat than broiling. Classic baked goods include breads, cookies, cakes, and savory dishes such as vegetarian lasagna and roasted vegetables. An example of using both techniques is when vegetarian lasagna is broiled after baking to melt a cheese topping or make the top crunchier. Baking typically is done for at least twenty minutes, whereas broiling is often done under ten minutes. Most ovens come equipped with a broiler. However, each oven is different. Broiling is done at a temperature of at least 500°F. You may need to leave your oven door slightly ajar while broiling. Refer to your owner's manual for more details.

A word about convection ovens: this option is ideal for cooking foods faster, being more energy-efficient, and cooking food more evenly than a regular oven. It also helps to brown foods (like roasted vegetables) while keeping their moisture inside. Convection works by blowing warm air over and around the food and cooks it quicker and more evenly. It is better for roasting; baking cakes, pies and cookies; or baking something covered with a top or cover. Use your regular oven setting, however, for delicate dishes such as custards and soufflés. Again, refer to your owner's manual for your specific oven recommendations.

LEARN HOW TO USE ALL OF YOUR APPLIANCES

I realize that you may not be as in love with your kitchen or its appliances as I am with mine. Perhaps you only venture into your kitchen by accident on your way to another room in your house, or maybe you have even considered converting it into storage for your shoes and pocketbooks. But another crucial step to creating vegan dishes is to make sure you understand how to use all of your appliances. They can be huge time-savers if used to their fullest potential. For example, your microwave may also have a convection oven setting. You may not realize what it is capable of until you read the manual. Also, you will be able to make adjustments in recipes according to how your appliances work. For example, if the instructions say to beat something on high for two minutes, your mixer could take longer if the "high" setting is not as powerful as the mixer used to test and write the original recipe. By exploring the options on my MultiPot, I recently discovered that there is no need to defrost a frozen chicken first. On a busy weeknight, that is a total time-saving game changer! And my MultiPot also makes delicious, belly-filling quinoa in just four minutes.

COMMON COOKING TERMS AND WHAT THEY MEAN

Once you get acquainted with your kitchen and start following and creating some recipes, you may come across some terms with which you are unfamiliar.

Here are some common terms you may encounter:

- *Mash*: This means to break down softened foods into smaller pieces while leaving them chunky or coarse. You can mash with a fork for smaller portions or use a masher tool like a potato masher. This is an easy way to make avocado toast with ripe avocados, for example. You may prefer to whip (either by hand or with a mixer) items that are normally mashed, such as potatoes or squash.
- *Whip*: This introduces air into something to make it lighter and fluffier. Batters and aquafaba are some examples. You can use a hand mixer, stand mixer, or a wire whisk to whip just about anything. In a pinch, a fork will work too.
- *Crush*: This is done to break down firm or hard items like ice. You can crush ingredients like garlic bulbs with the back of your knife, your palm, or other heavy objects. There are also special kitchen gadgets used for crushing.
- *Grate*: This technique breaks down solid food into small, fine pieces. Graters come in different forms. To grate an orange or lemon peel, ginger, or garlic, a small handheld grater or Microplane is best.
- *Blend*: This is a way to combine a variety of solid and liquid items. The final product can be smooth or have a slight texture to it. Blending is typically done with cold food or beverages and may include ice. Depending on what you are blending, you have three choices: a regular blender, a handheld immersion blender (works best for soups), and a food processor. The tool you should use will depend on the recipe.
- *Puree:* This technique is similar to blending, but the final product is usually smooth and creamy liquid. Also, pureeing tends to be used for warm foods. When a recipe tells you to puree something, you can do it in small batches in a regular blender, an immersion blender, or in a food processor.

This is just an overview of some of the techniques you will encounter. A good, comprehensive cookbook will help you define any other terms you need to learn—and of course, there is always Chef Google.

Chapter 4:
CREATING A COMPLETE MEAL

TRUE OR FALSE: All vegans are at their ideal body weights and are super healthy.

FALSE: It is still possible to eat too many bad calories as a vegan, despite the wealth of healthier options from which they can choose. Vegans have to create balanced meals from quality sources. This can be a challenge, especially for new vegans. For example, certain vitamins and minerals, such as vitamin B12 and iron, are more easily found in meat products, so finding plant sources for these just requires doing a little exploring.

NUTRITIONAL CONSIDERATIONS

This section will cover some of the challenges many vegans face when putting meals together. It is designed to help you create healthy and balanced meal combinations that will leave you full of energy and health. If you want to lose weight or maintain your ideal body weight, just remember not to consume too many empty calories in addition. Keep your exercise regimen consistent and challenging, and stay hydrated!

GETTING ADEQUATE PROTEIN

TRUE OR FALSE: You can get enough protein and build muscle only by eating meat.

FALSE: The largest animal on dry land, the elephant, is a vegan. Other large vegan animals include gorillas, horses, cows, rhinos, and bison. Not exactly wispy little things, are they?

Unless they look like Dwayne Johnson, aka the Rock, most carnivores may not give much thought to getting enough protein. They can easily get what they need from dairy products and a serving or two of meat or fish. But vegans need to get all of their protein from plant sources.

Fortunately, there are many options in the plant world that are rich in protein:

- Soy products such as edamame, tofu, and tempeh
- Nuts, nut milks, nut butters, and seeds (pumpkin, chia, and flax)

- Grains, especially quinoa, oats, and whole wheat
- Legumes such as kidney beans, lentils, and chickpeas

GETTING ENOUGH IRON

Some vegans and vegetarians may be iron deficient, but this could be due to medical problems, such as heavy menstrual periods in women or intestinal issues that affect iron absorption, rather than their diet. The iron in plant sources (non-heme iron) is not absorbed as well as the iron from animal sources (heme) is absorbed. To make the iron from plant protein more absorbable, you should pair it with vitamin C-rich foods (citrus fruits, bell peppers, melons, and strawberries) or beverages. For example, drinking a small glass of orange juice with a meal that contains a lot of iron-rich foods will increase the amount of iron that is absorbed. Beta-carotene, which your body turns into vitamin A, also helps with the absorption of iron. Beta-carotene is found in foods that are red or orange-colored, such as sweet potatoes, carrots, red peppers, oranges, peaches, cantaloupe, squash, and dark leafy greens like spinach and kale. In the meantime, you can boost your iron intake by eating these foods:

- Dark leafy greens, such as spinach
- Green beans
- Wheat germ
- Lima beans, kidney beans, or chickpeas
- Dried fruit such as raisins, apricots, and prunes
- Lentils
- Blackstrap molasses (can be used in baking or taken as a supplement)
- Pumpkin, squash, or sesame seeds
- Iron-enriched breakfast cereals
- Peanuts, pecans, walnuts, etc.

Cooking in a cast-iron skillet may help increase the iron in your food. Some sources support this claim; others do not. If you are using a "seasoned" skillet (one that has a nice sheen from being baked with oil or used repeatedly), this is less likely to happen because of the coating developed over time, making it less reactive with your food. Studies have shown that cooking in a cast-iron skillet may raise your blood iron levels somewhat, but more research is needed.[3]

Other factors to consider include what kind of food is being cooked, how long it is being cooked, your age, and even how old the pot itself is.

America's Test Kitchen made a comparison to see how much iron was released from simmering tomato sauce in a stainless-steel pan, a seasoned cast-iron pan, and an unseasoned one. While the levels of iron were the highest in the tomato sauce made in the unseasoned pan, the amounts of iron that were released from both the seasoned cast-iron skillet and the stainless-steel pan were essentially the same. Since most people do not use an *unseasoned* cast-iron skillet for cooking, this would not seem to be a major contributor of iron to your meals. In fact, as I sit here typing this, I am re-seasoning my "ashy" cast-iron skillets. To do this, all I did was make sure my skillets (yes, I have three) were clean and dry. I then wiped them down with canola oil and placed them in the oven to bake upside down for 1 hour at 450°F. I covered the lower rack with aluminum foil to catch any drippings. I then turned the oven off and let them remain in the oven to cool off. You can also just place them in the oven and run the self-clean cycle. It is good to season your cast-iron at least twice a year. By doing so, you maintain the natural nonstick surface and prevent it from rusting.

Be aware that drinking coffee and tea can actually *decrease* your iron absorption. Calcium can also negatively affect your iron absorption, so do not mix your iron-rich and calcium-rich foods together.

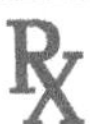
DOCTOR'S ORDERS

If you are concerned that your iron levels are low, your doctor can check your iron levels and tell you if you need to boost your intake or even prescribe iron replacements for you.

FINDING FOODS RICH IN B VITAMINS

Vegans get most of their B vitamins from grains. B vitamins help your body make energy, produce red blood cells, and keep your brain and nervous system healthy. The B vitamins are:

- B1 (thiamine)
- B2 (riboflavin)
- B3 (niacin)
- B5 (pantothenic acid)
- B6 (pyridoxine)

- B7 (biotin)
- B9 (folate; used to produce folic acid)
- B12 (cobalamin)

Vitamin B12 is found in beef and poultry, but vegans can get an adequate supply from vitamin B12-fortified nutritional yeast, fortified cereals, fortified soy, tempeh, mushrooms, algae, and seaweed.

GETTING ENOUGH CALCIUM

In addition to natural sources of calcium, fortified foods are another way for vegans to get enough calcium. The average recommended daily amount is 1000 milligrams (mg). Some foods that are calcium-rich include:

- Soy milks, nut milks, and rice milks: they should contain at least 240 mg of calcium per 6.5–7 ounces.
- Nuts such as hazelnuts and almonds
- Leafy green vegetables and other vegetables such as bok choy, collard greens, turnip greens, and okra
- Beans, peas, and lentils
- Seeds, such as chia and flax

When preparing your vegetables, try not to boil them unless you will use the water as well (I love the taste of my mother's "pot liquor": the liquid left over from cooking collard, mustard, or turnip greens). A lot of the calcium, B vitamins, and C vitamins leave the food during the cooking process and can be lost in the water (known as "leaching"). The best way to preserve those healthy nutrients is to steam, stir-fry, or roast your veggies. Microwaving actually preserves delicate nutrients such as vitamin C due to the shorter cooking time involved.

PUTTING IT ALL TOGETHER

If you have been a vegan for a while, you probably already have the hang of this. If not, you may want to map some of your meals out in advance until meal planning becomes second nature to you. Even if you are not new to a vegan diet, it may be a good idea to take a step back, re-evaluate, and plan a few meals using new ingredients from time to time. Not only will this help ensure that you get the nutrients you need, but it helps build variety because you will learn how to use new ingredients in your meal planning.

Besides planning meals, keep a food journal. Use it to keep track of what you eat, how you cooked it, whether you liked it, and if you would change anything. A food journal is also a good way to see if you are getting the right nutrients. Don't get analysis paralysis: use your journal to get a gestalt of your diet. Simply peruse it to make sure you are getting what you need. Use it as a road map on your lifelong journey of health! Remember, it is impossible to know where you are going if you do not remember where you have been and how you got there.

VEGAN-FRIENDLY ETHNIC CUISINE

While your vegan journey may just be beginning, keep in mind that there are various ethnic cuisines that have offered vegan and vegetarian fare for centuries. As a result, they have a lot of tasty vegan dishes that you can enjoy. This gives your diet much-needed variety and takes the guesswork out of it for you. Familiarize yourself with the many different options from around the globe. No need to reinvent the wheel. If you live in a culturally diverse area like a major city, venture out and try something new (if your budget allows for it). If not, go to Chef Google and see what you can make at home.

Below is a list of international cuisines to try. Most of these also have meat dishes, but their vegetarian options are delicious as well.

- ***Indian:*** includes grain and vegetable-based options.
- ***Chinese:*** look for vegetarian options on the menu.
- ***Korean:*** features rice and vegetable dishes.
- ***Thai:*** similar to traditional, produce-based Chinese food, Thai food uses more herbs and spices and packs some heat.
- ***Vietnamese:*** another Asian cuisine that uses a lot of plant-based foods.
- ***Greek:*** Mediterranean cuisine in general is vegan-friendly because there are a lot of dishes that feature plant-based foods and healthy fats like omega-3 fatty acids. The vegan parts of the "Mediterranean diet" include fruits, vegetables, nuts, seeds, legumes, whole grains, herbs, and extra-virgin olive oil.

℞ DOCTOR'S NOTES

Just about any dish can be "vegan-ized," for example, my ***Cauliflower Rice Stir-Fry with Duck Sauce and Hot Mustard*** *recipe, made entirely with plant-based sources. I substituted tofu for the scrambled eggs, and I used cauliflower rice to cut back on carbs. It is just as flavorful as the "real" thing!*

Chapter 5:

SPECIAL NUTRITIONAL CONSIDERATIONS

The vegan diet is ideal for helping you live your best life! As mentioned previously, however, it is still possible for vegans to be overweight due to excessive intake of junk calories. Vegans can also be unhealthy if they do not get enough of the right nutrients. However, these problems can be easily fixed by choosing the right calories and creating more complete meals.

But some people have additional health problems to consider. Some may be trying a vegan diet to help restore their health. Others may choose to become vegan for other reasons, like concern for the environment, and it just so happens they also have health problems like diabetes. Adopting a vegan lifestyle may prevent the development of some of these conditions, especially if you have a family history.

Let's look at some common health conditions and how to adjust the vegan diet to accommodate them. Remember, the vegan diet is a healthy diet to begin with, so making these adjustments should be relatively easy.

℞ DOCTOR'S ORDERS

As a reminder, this information is not meant to prevent, diagnose, treat, or cure any disease. You should consult your personal physician before making any changes to your diet.

DIABETES

Diabetes is a condition that results in high blood sugar. For the most part, there are two types of diabetes. Type 1, which is usually diagnosed in childhood and associated with weight loss, is caused by a lack of insulin and can be life-threatening. Type 2, typically diagnosed in adulthood, is caused by insulin resistance (your body has enough insulin, but your organs do not respond to it as they should). Type 2 diabetes commonly results in weight gain and is usually not life-threatening. The vegan diet, being low-fat and low in sugar, is especially useful for people who have type 2 diabetes. However, type 1 sufferers can also benefit. The prediabetic condition known as insulin resistance can also benefit from a vegan diet. If you stick to low-fat foods, whole foods, whole grains, legumes, nuts, seeds, and plenty of fruits and vegetables, it will help manage your condition naturally. Work with your doctor and dietician to understand how the glycemic index works so you can avoid wide swings in your blood sugar levels. The glycemic index (GI) is a measure of how slowly or quickly, or how high, your blood sugar rises after you eat. Some foods have a larger impact on your blood sugar than others. An ideal GI score is less than 55. Foods such as fruits, vegetables, nuts, beans, and whole grains are in this category. High GI foods include white bread, bagels, baked goods (doughnuts and cakes), croissants, and most crackers. If you have diabetes, be sure to take your medication as prescribed.

DISEASES OF THE CIRCULATORY SYSTEM

The cardiovascular system includes your heart and blood vessels (arteries, veins, and capillaries). Diseases of the cardiovascular system, such as high cholesterol, high blood pressure, and coronary artery disease, can all be improved by a vegan diet since it is low in fat and cholesterol. Avoid consuming excess sodium or salt if you have hypertension (high blood pressure). Keep your daily intake to less than 2000 mg, which is less than a teaspoon of table salt. Following a vegan diet benefits your health and can help with these health problems. Using fresh herbs and spices to season your food and reducing your sodium intake will help control your blood pressure as well. Aim for a blood pressure of less than 120/80 unless your doctor tells you otherwise.

LOW-FAT DIET

As we have seen, the vegan diet is naturally low in bad fats. Because no animal products are being consumed, the diet is low in saturated fat and high in the helpful fats that come from avocadoes, nuts, seeds, and various vegetable oils. Remember to avoid trans fats. They raise your bad cholesterol (LDL) and lower your good cholesterol (HDL). This increases your heart attack risk. Trans fats also may raise the risk for diabetes. Therefore, they are worse for you than saturated fats. A small amount of saturated fat in your diet may be okay, and it can even raise your good cholesterol. No more than 10 percent of your total daily calories should come from saturated fats. One source of saturated fat is coconut, which can be eaten occasionally. Cooking with coconut oil instead of butter or lard is another option.

LOW-SODIUM COOKING

People who follow the vegan diet can consume too much sodium just like anyone else. Followed in its purest state, the vegan diet is low in sodium. But reach for the saltshaker too often, and this could negatively affect your health. Packaged and processed foods are available whether you are vegan or not. Avoid them and the saltshaker, especially if you tend to retain water or have high blood pressure. Again, experiment with different herbs and spices to enhance the flavor of your food. Different cooking techniques, such as grilling, baking, and air frying can also enhance the natural flavor of food.

GLUTEN-FREE COOKING

Gluten is a protein found in grains such as rye, barley, and wheat. For most people, it causes no ill effects. But for a small percentage of people, gluten causes a wide range of symptoms, including skin rashes, diarrhea, headache, joint pain, and fatigue. Symptoms can be mild (gluten sensitivity) or severe (celiac disease). At first glance, it may seem like a challenge to avoid gluten on a vegan diet. However, it is still very possible. Here is a short list of some of the grains to avoid:

- Barley
- Wheat
- Rye
- Spelt

However, there are still plenty of grains and starches that people with gluten sensitivity can eat:

- Oats
- Rice, especially brown rice
- Quinoa
- Corn
- Millet
- Amaranth
- Potatoes
- Beer made from these grains instead of wheat or barley

Just follow the vegan diet as you would normally and incorporate gluten-free options.

Keep in mind that there are many other conditions that can be improved by a vegan diet. These are just a few of the more common examples. As you can see, the vegan diet can be easily adapted to help with a variety of health problems. The only limit is your imagination!

I don't know about you, but after talking about all this food, I am getting hungry! Let's meet in the kitchen, shall we?

Disclaimer: The amounts of salt I use throughout this book may be less than what you prefer. As with any recipe, season to taste (but go easy on that salt, folks).

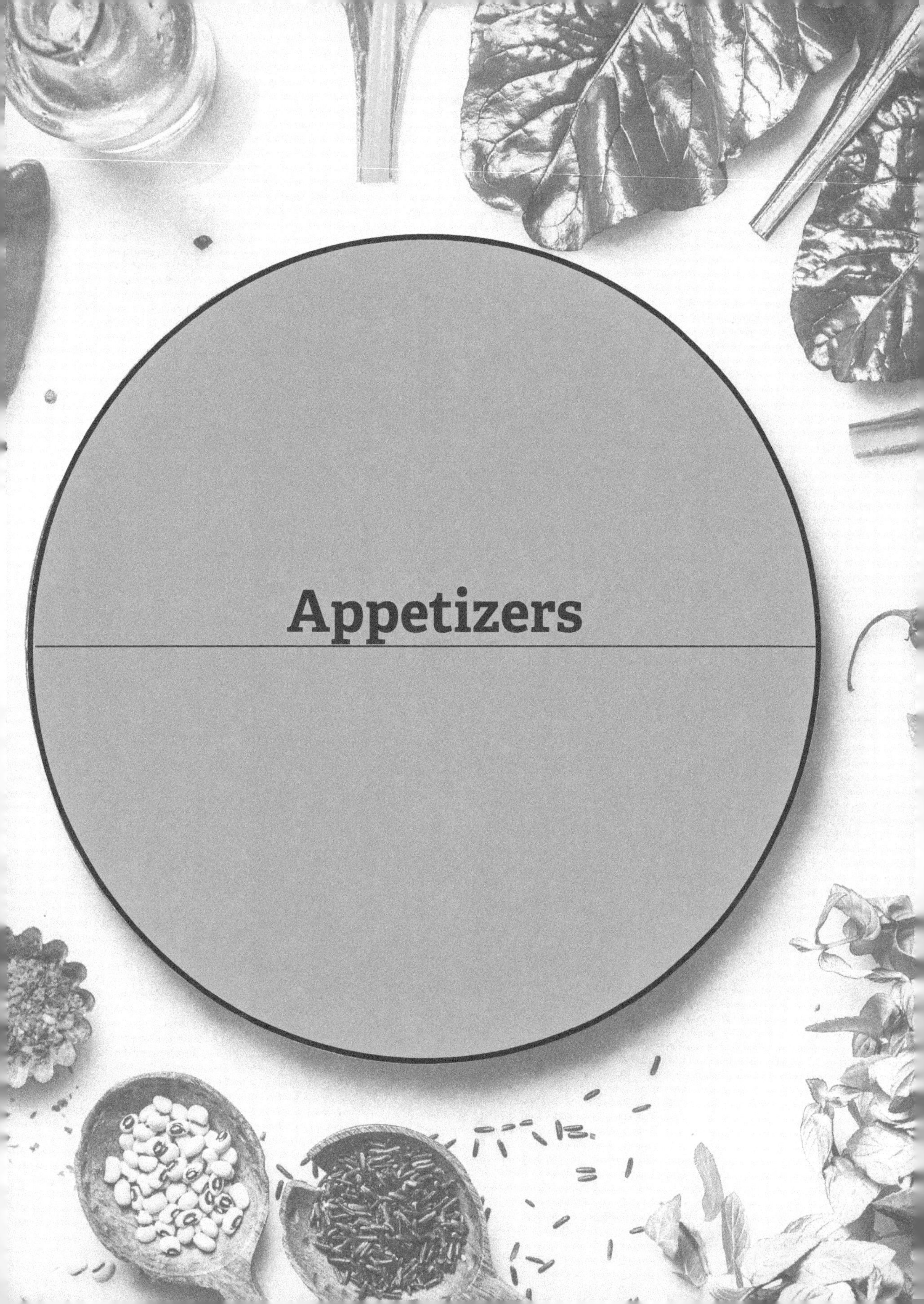

Appetizers

Vegan appetizers can be super easy to make and are a nutritious way to fill up on veggies before the main course, which will help you control your portion sizes during the entrée and dessert portions of the meal.

BLACK OLIVE HUMMUS

Hummus is a classic vegan food that is low in fat and high in protein. Spread this on whole grain vegan crackers or serve with bread. The olives provide the salt in this recipe.

- 1 (15-ounce) can cooked chickpeas, drained and rinsed
- ½ cup tahini
- 1 tablespoon water
- ⅓ cup fresh lemon juice
- ¼ cup pitted black olives, diced
- 4 garlic cloves, peeled and ends removed
- ½–1 cup extra virgin olive oil, more as needed

Combine all the ingredients except the olive oil in a food processor or blender and pulse until creamy. With the motor running, drizzle in the olive oil until the mixture is thick and creamy. Transfer to a serving dish and serve with crackers, bread, or whole grain pita wedges.

Makes 2–4 servings.

GRILLED VEGETABLE SKEWERS

- 1 medium zucchini, cut into 1-inch-thick rounds
- 1 medium yellow squash, cut into 1-inch-thick rounds
- 1 red or orange bell pepper, sliced
- 1 pound button or cremini mushrooms, cleaned and stems cut off
- 2 red onions, cut into thick slices
- 1–2 tablespoons oil for grilling, such as avocado or sunflower oil
- Salt and pepper to taste

Preheat a grill on medium heat. Place all vegetable pieces in a large bowl, drizzle with oil, and season with a healthy pinch of salt and pepper. Using a skewer (metal or wooden), thread the vegetable pieces from top to bottom. Alternate for color, size, and variety until all pieces have been used. Grill for 5–7 minutes on each side until the desired grill marks and tenderness are reached. Serve warm. Drizzle with the **Vegan Green Goddess Dressing.**

Makes 4 servings.

Notes: Wooden skewers should be soaked for 20–30 minutes before use to prevent burning or scorching. Metal skewers do not need to be soaked, but to avoid burns, use heat-resistant gloves.

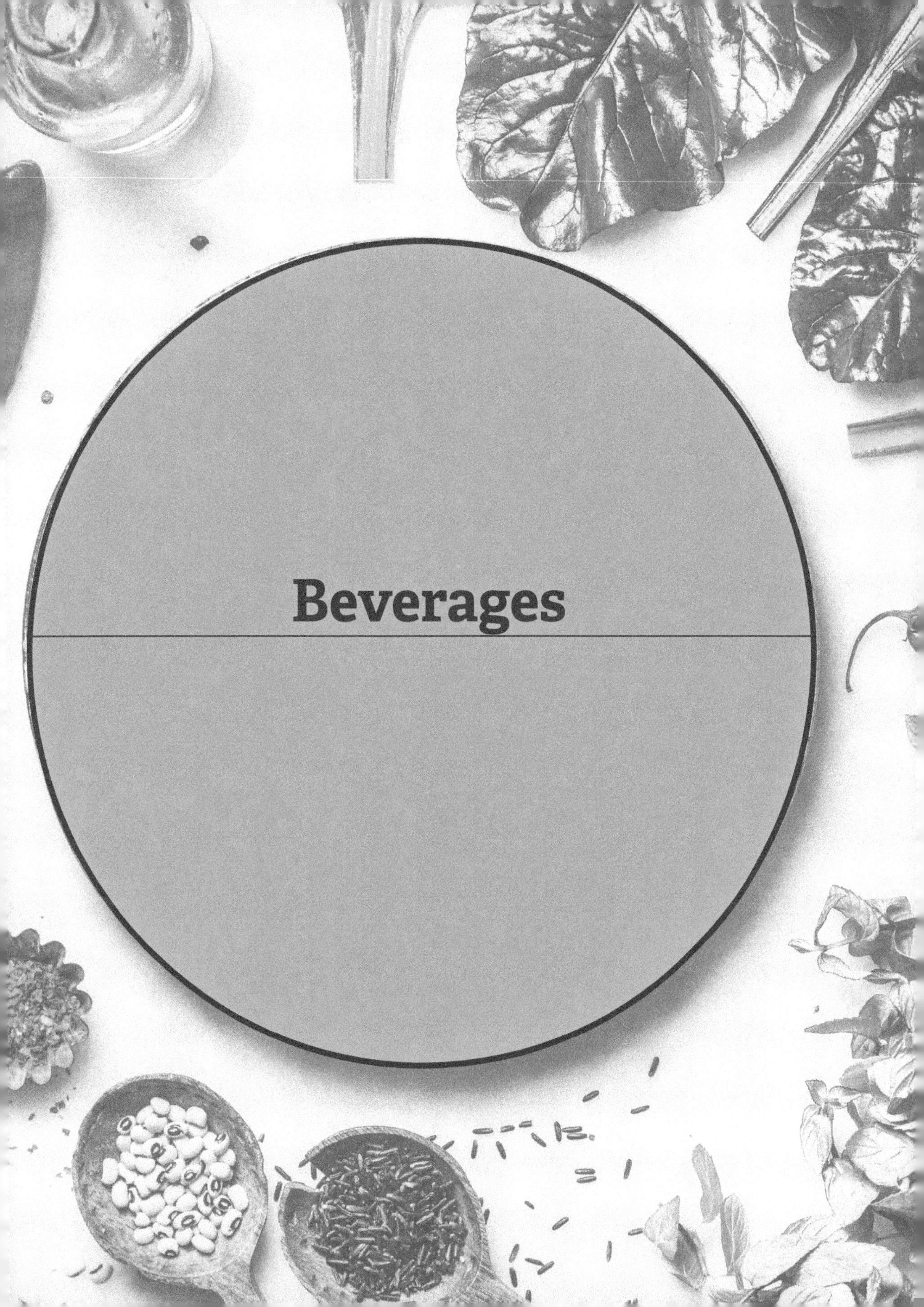

Beverages

These drinks can be made to go with any meal or just to hydrate throughout the day.

DR. MONIQUE'S MANGO MUDDLED MINT MOCK MO-GARITA

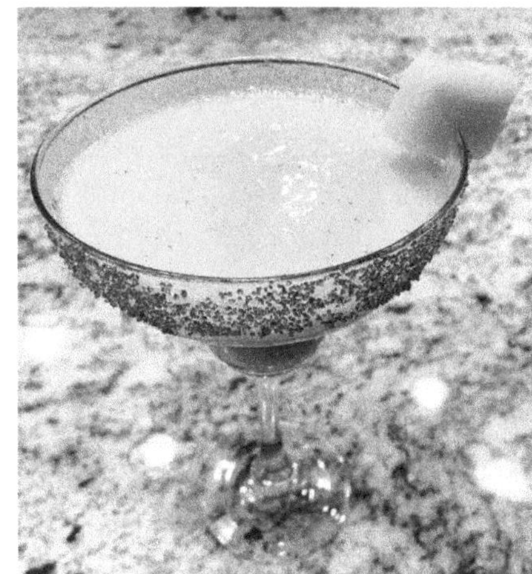

- 1 cup frozen mango
- ½ cup frozen pineapple
- 3–4 mint leaves
- Juice of 1 lime
- ½ cup coconut water
- ½ cup lime sparkling water
- Coarse salt, lime zest, or green sugar for rimming (optional)
- Pineapple rings or chunks for garnish (optional)
- Lime wedges for garnish (optional)

Place a margarita glass in the freezer for 15–20 minutes. Place all ingredients except the garnishes in a blender and puree until smooth. Place lime zest, salt, or sugar in a small plate. Rub outside of glass with a lime wedge. Roll the rim of the glass in the plate to make an even edge. Rim only the outside of the glass to avoid getting salt in your drink. Pour the Mo-garita in the margarita glass and garnish with pineapple or lime wedge.

Makes 2 servings.

LEMON, GINGER, AND BASIL WATER

- 2 large or 4 small lemons, sliced
- ½-inch knob ginger, grated finely
- ¼ cup fresh basil, roughly chopped

Add all ingredients to a water bottle or pitcher with 64 ounces of water and shake or mix well. Add ice cubes as desired. Strain the water through a fine-mesh strainer to remove large particles if desired.

Makes 6–8 servings.

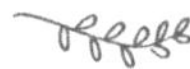

HOMEMADE ORANGE JUICE

- 2 navel oranges, peeled
- 4–6 kiwis, peeled ½ cantaloupe, cut into chunks
- 2 Gala apples, cored and sliced
- 1 cup pineapple, peeled and cut into cubes (optional)
- ½-inch knob fresh ginger

Place the pieces of fruit and ginger into an electric juicer. Juice the ingredients per your juicer's operating manual instructions. I start and finish with the softer fruits like kiwi to help flush out the juicer. Drink immediately or store in the refrigerator in a glass jar with a tight lid for up to 48 hours. This stops the oxidation of the vitamins and keeps your juice potent.

Makes 4 servings.

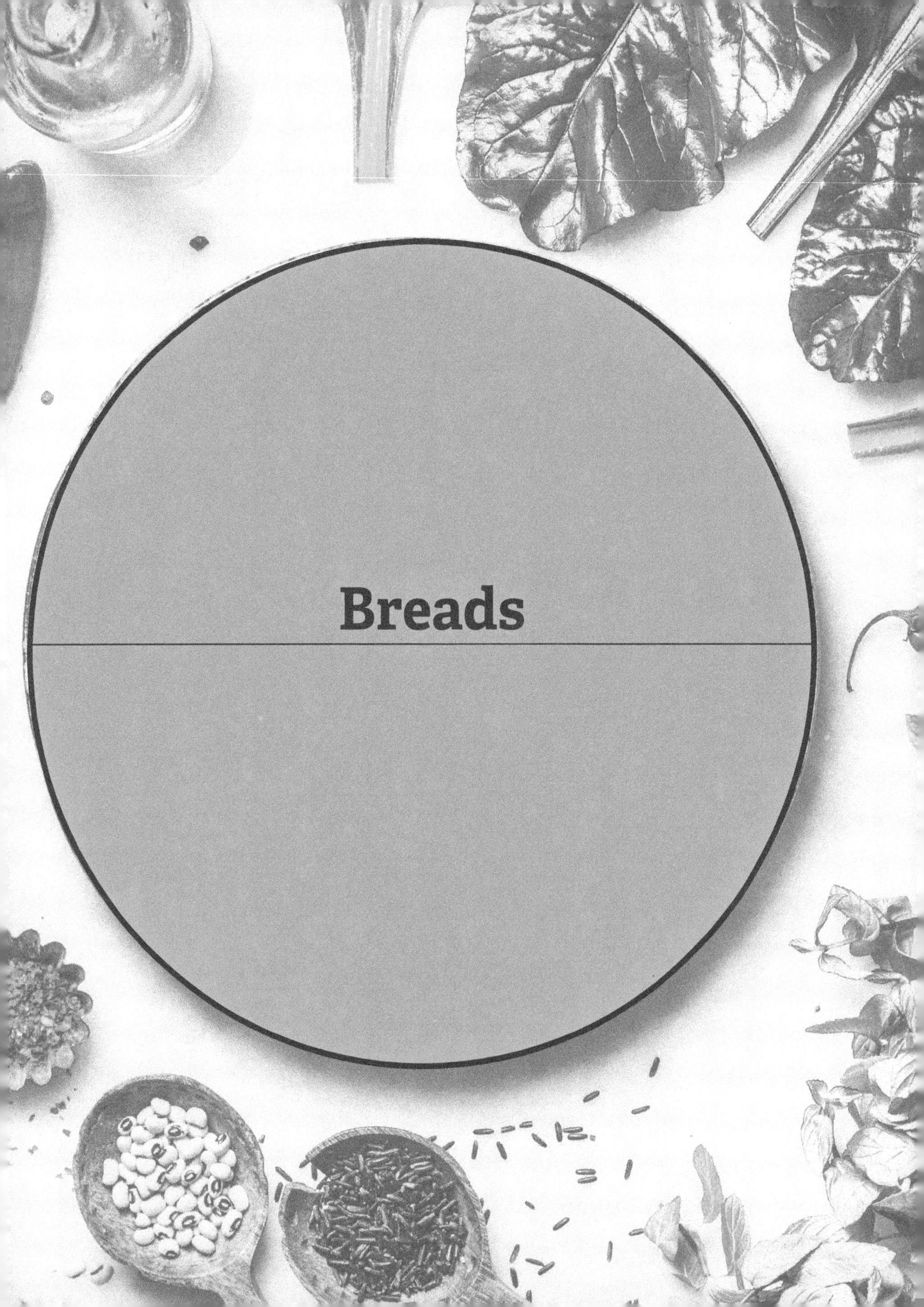

Breads

Not all bread is bad for you! And you do not have to own a fancy bread maker to make it at home.

VEGAN CORNBREAD

- 1½ cups cornmeal
- ½ cup whole wheat flour
- 1 tablespoon sugar
- 1 teaspoon kosher salt
- 2 teaspoons baking powder
- 1 cup vegan buttermilk*
- 6 tablespoons aquafaba
- 1 stick plant butter, melted and divided into 1 tablespoon and 7 tablespoons

Preheat the oven to 400°F. Place a cast-iron skillet in the oven to heat while you make the cornbread batter. Using a whisk or a fork, mix all the dry ingredients in a large bowl. Then whisk in the vegan buttermilk, aquafaba, and 7 of the 8 tablespoons of melted butter. Decrease the oven temperature to 400°F. Use an oven mitt to remove the skillet from the oven. Coat the skillet pan with the remaining tablespoon of melted butter. Add the batter to the skillet and bake 20–25 minutes until the surface is golden brown and crusty or firm to the touch. Serve warm with butter and jelly or maple syrup.

*Notes: If you do not have buttermilk, add 1 teaspoon of vinegar to 1 cup of plant milk and mix well. Let sit for 10 minutes until curdled.

Makes 6–8 servings.

VEGAN ZUCCHINI BREAD

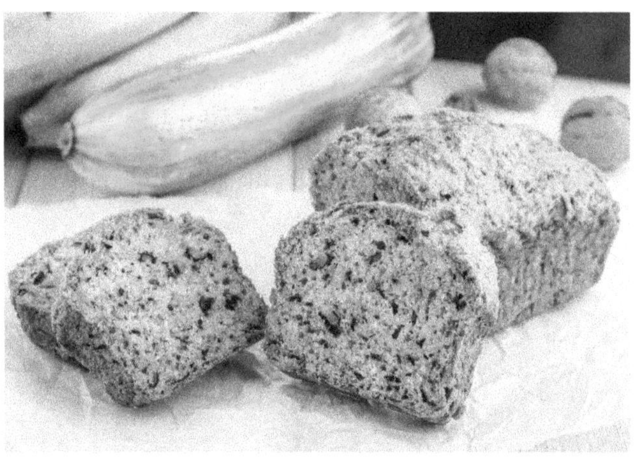

- 2 tablespoons ground flaxseed
- 6 tablespoons water
- 1 large zucchini, grated
- 2 cups gluten-free flour
- 1 cup coconut sugar
- 2 teaspoons cinnamon
- ½ teaspoon nutmeg
- ½ teaspoon ground cardamom
- ½ teaspoon salt
- 2 teaspoons baking powder
- 1½ teaspoons baking soda
- ½ cup coconut oil, melted
- ½ cup organic applesauce
- 2 teaspoons vanilla
- 1½ tablespoons apple cider vinegar
- ½ cup walnuts, toasted and crushed

Preheat the oven to 350°F. Spray a loaf pan with nonstick spray. Whisk the flaxseed and water in a small bowl and place in the refrigerator for 10 minutes (the mixture should be the consistency of an egg yolk). Roughly chop the zucchini into large chunks and place in a food processor (peeling is not necessary). Use the grating attachment to grate or shred (use a box grater if you don't have a food processor). Wrap the grated zucchini in a clean kitchen towel and wring out as much liquid as you can before placing it in a large bowl. In another bowl, whisk together flour, sugar, cinnamon, nutmeg, cardamom, salt, baking powder, and baking soda in a large bowl. Add the grated zucchini, coconut oil, applesauce, vanilla, and apple cider vinegar to another bowl and mix well. Add the wet ingredients to the dry ingredients and stir with a spoon until well-blended. The batter will be thick. Add most of the walnuts and stir until just blended in. Add the batter to the loaf pan and sprinkle with more walnuts. Bake for 60–70 minutes, until a toothpick inserted in the center comes out clean. Let the bread cool in the pan for 10–15 minutes, then remove and let cool for another 30 minutes on a wire rack.

Makes 6–8 servings.

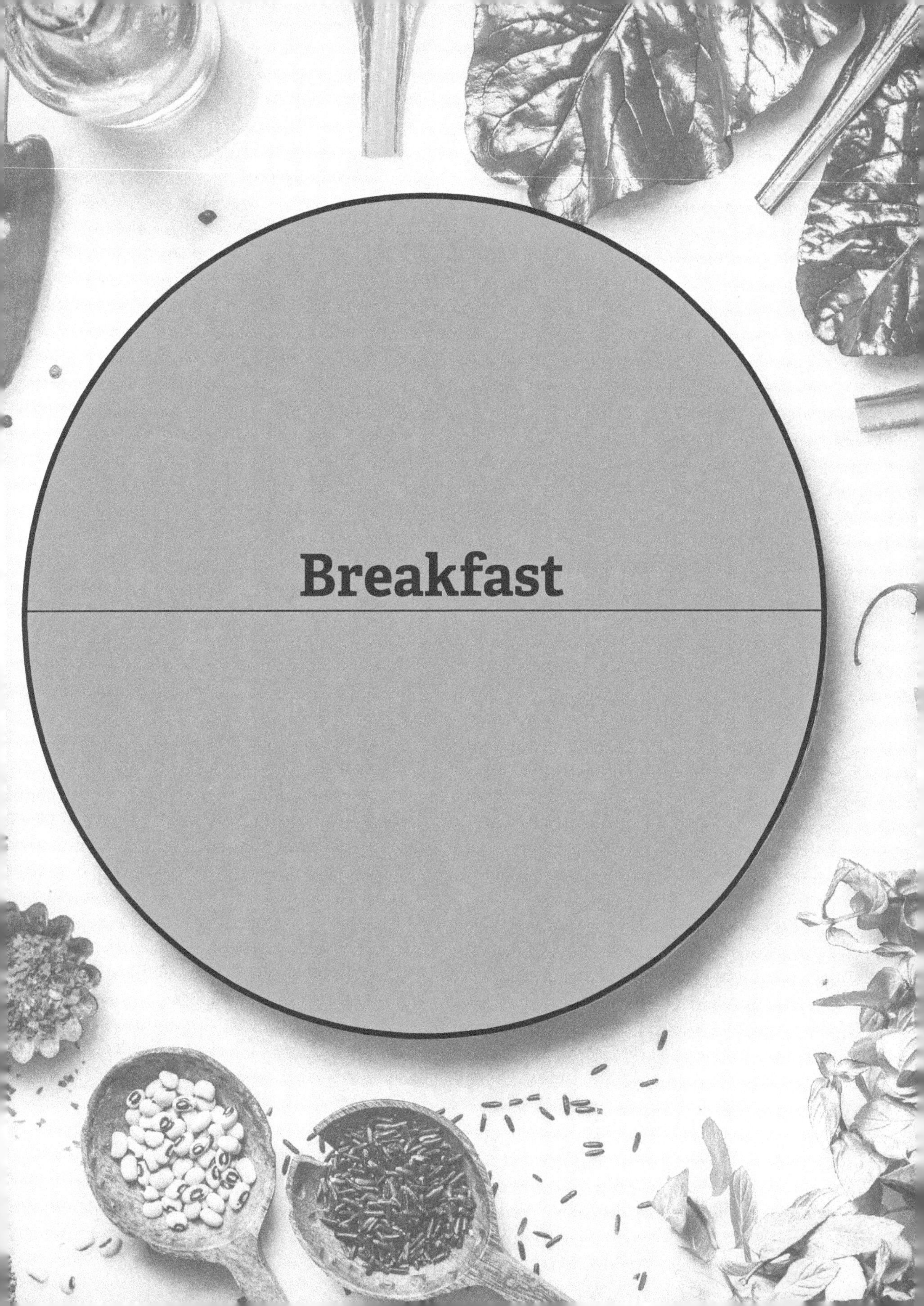

Breakfast

The following recipes are my take on some breakfast classics, using ingredients we may typically think of using for lunch or dinner. It is so important to start the day off with a belly full of good fats, fiber, protein, vitamins, and minerals.

AVOCADO WAFFLES

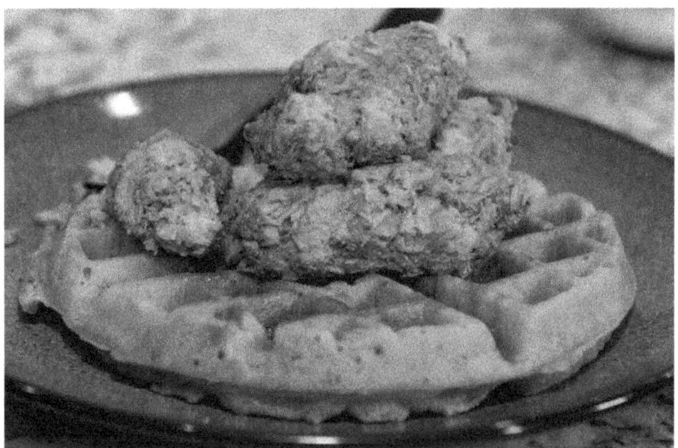

- 2 cups whole wheat flour
- ¼ cup organic confectioners' sugar
- 2 teaspoons baking powder
- ½ teaspoon salt
- ¼ teaspoon baking soda
- 1 teaspoon cumin
- 1½ cups almond milk
- 1½ sticks plant butter, melted
- 2 ripe avocados, mashed well with a fork
- ¼ cup chopped fresh cilantro
- 100-percent maple syrup for topping
- Plant butter for topping

In a large bowl, whisk all the dry ingredients together. In a separate bowl, mix the wet ingredients, including the avocados. Add the chopped fresh cilantro to the wet ingredients and combine well. Pour the wet mixture into the dry mixture and stir until just combined. A few small lumps are fine. Preheat a waffle iron; spray with nonstick spray, and then fill the waffle iron three-quarters full with batter and cook until the waffles are golden and crisp. Do not overfill the waffle iron. Serve warm and top with plant butter, more chopped cilantro, chick'n (see below), and 100-percent maple syrup.

Chick'n

I use a plant-based chicken mix that I order from Australia called Deliciou to make my chick'n tenders in my air fryer, but you can use chicken or any plant-based replacement you prefer. Cook the chick'n according to the package directions.

Makes 3–4 waffles.

CHOCOLATE QUINOA

This bowl of warm, yummy goodness is like eating dessert for breakfast! The chocolate lovers in your house will love it. How do I know? Because it got the thumbs-up from the chocolate eater in my house: my son, Mitchell!

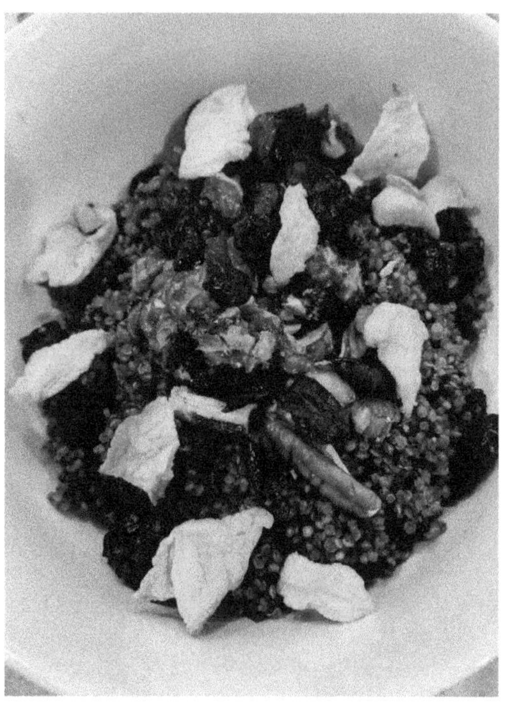

- 1 cup quinoa, rinsed
- 1¼ cups almond milk
- 1 tablespoon unsweetened Dutch cocoa powder
- 1 teaspoon vanilla
- ¼ teaspoon kosher salt
- ¼ cup maple syrup
- Dried cranberries and apple slices for topping
- Toasted pecans or walnuts for topping

Add all ingredients to a multicooker such as a Power Quick Pot or an Instant Pot and cook using the quinoa setting. Allow to sit for 5–10 minutes when done. Fluff with a fork. Top with your favorite toppings and enjoy while still warm. If using a pressure cooker, cook on high for 1–3 minutes and then allow the pressure to release gradually for 8–10 minutes. If cooking on the stovetop, add all of the ingredients to a medium-sized pot and follow the package directions to cook the quinoa. Fluff with a fork before serving, and top with dried fruits and toasted nuts.

Makes 4–6 servings.

SWEET POTATO HASH

I made this with frozen sweet potato fries, but you can substitute with fresh sweet potatoes instead if you wish. If you want to use fresh herbs, you can substitute those as well. Just remember that 1 teaspoon of dried herbs equals 1 tablespoon of fresh herbs. For meat-eaters, turkey sausage crumbles can be added, or to keep the recipe strictly vegan, tofu or plant-based meat substitutes can be a nice addition. Either way, you will have a flavorful, belly-filling hash with more health benefits than white potatoes. Also, broiling this in your skillet is an extra step that dries the potatoes out just enough and adds a bit of crispiness.

- 2–3 tablespoons olive oil
- 1 red onion, diced
- 2 large bell peppers (green, yellow, red, or orange), diced
- 1–2 teaspoons minced garlic
- 4 cups loosely packed frozen sweet potato fries, thawed and diced
- 2 teaspoons smoked paprika
- ½ teaspoon chili powder
- 1 teaspoon dried thyme
- 1 teaspoon dried rosemary
- 1 teaspoon salt
- ½ teaspoon ground black pepper
- Fresh parsley for garnish, chopped

Using a large cast-iron skillet, swirl olive oil into the skillet and warm over medium heat. Add the onion and peppers and cook until just tender, about 3–5 minutes. Add the garlic and cook for about 30–60 seconds until fragrant. Add the sweet potatoes, smoked paprika, chili powder, thyme, rosemary, salt, and black pepper, and cook for 15 minutes or until the potatoes are warm and slightly browned, stirring frequently.

Optional: Spread the hash evenly over the skillet and broil in a preheated oven at 450°F for an additional 8–10 minutes until the potatoes are a bit crispy and serve warm. Top with fresh parsley.

Makes 6–8 servings.

HANDFUL SMOOTHIE

- 1 handful of fresh spinach
- 1 handful of frozen berries
- 1 handful of frozen riced cauliflower
- 2 tablespoons vegan or Greek yogurt
- 1 cup almond milk or coconut water
- 1 heaping tablespoon ground flaxseed
- 1 scoop of vegan protein powder (optional)

Combine all the ingredients in a blender until smooth. Drink immediately.

Optional add-ins: honey, ground cinnamon, vanilla flavoring, 100-percent fruit juice, or frozen fruit of your choice.

Makes 1 smoothie.

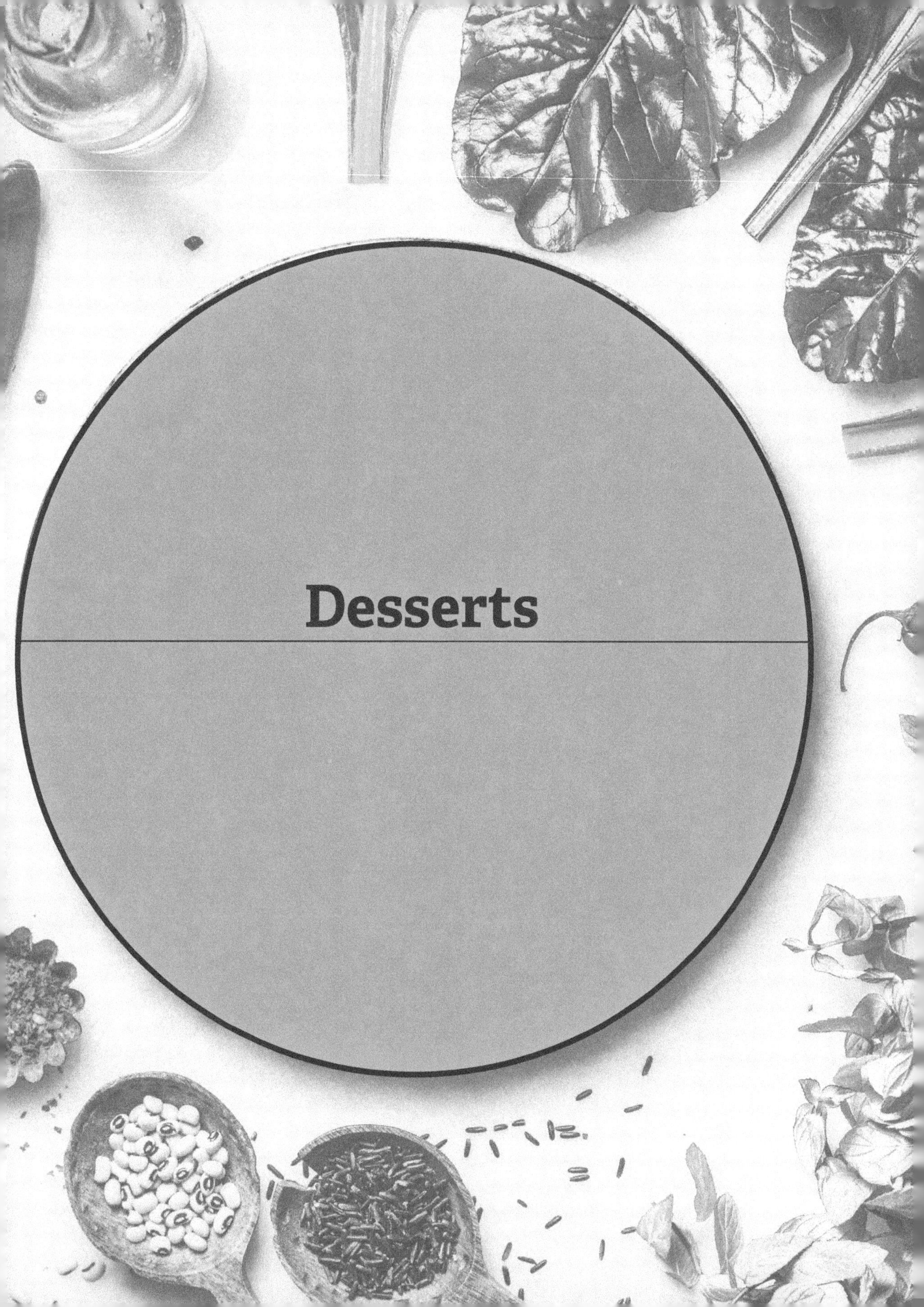

Desserts

MITCHELL'S VEGAN AND GLUTEN-FREE CHOCOLATE CAKE

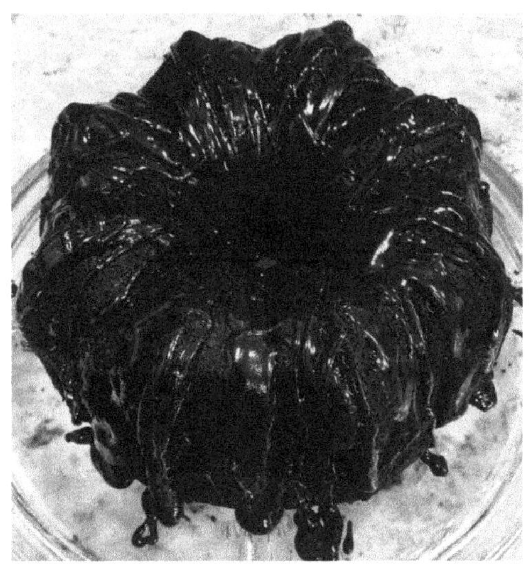

- 2 tablespoons finely ground flaxseed*
- ½ cup plus 6 tablespoons water
- 2½ cups gluten-free flour
- 1 cup unsweetened Dutch cocoa powder
- 1 teaspoon baking powder
- 2 teaspoons baking soda
- ½ teaspoon salt
- 1 cup almond or soy milk
- 1 cup coconut oil, melted and cooled
- 2 tablespoons apple cider vinegar
- 2 teaspoons vanilla
- 2 cups maple syrup

Preheat the oven to 350°F. Spray a nonstick 10-inch Bundt pan with nonstick spray. Make 2 fleggs: Mix the flaxseed and 6 tablespoons of water until combined and refrigerate for 10–15 minutes. The mixture should have an egg yolk-like consistency. Sift all the dry ingredients together in one bowl. Add the milk, coconut oil, apple cider vinegar, vanilla, maple syrup, and ½ cup water to another bowl and combine. Add the wet ingredients to the dry ingredients and mix until well-incorporated. Stir in the flegg mixture. Do not overmix the batter. Bake for 40–45 minutes or until an inserted toothpick comes out dry. Let cool in the pan for 10 minutes, then invert the pan onto a cake plate and allow to cool completely before drizzling the **Chocolate Glaze** (see recipe) over it. Store the cake covered at cool room temperature for 3–5 days. Keep refrigerated if the room temperature is warm.

Makes 14–16 servings.

NOTES FROM THE LAB

Make your own finely ground flaxseed: place ground flaxseed in a spice grinder and process until finely ground. If you do not have a spice grinder, a coffee grinder, pepper mill, or mortar and pestle will work as well.

Chocolate Glaze

- ¼ cup coconut milk
- ½ cup vegan semisweet chocolate chips
- 2 teaspoons vanilla
- 1 teaspoon maple syrup

> **NOTES FROM THE LAB**
>
> You can also use 4 ounces of silken tofu instead of coconut milk. Be sure to drain the tofu first so that your glaze won't be too runny.
>
> Makes about 1 cup.

Place the milk and chocolate chips in a microwave-safe bowl. Microwave in 15–30 second intervals until melted. Stir with a spatula after every 15 seconds. Add in the vanilla and maple syrup and stir until combined. Drizzle over the cooled **Vegan & Gluten-Free Chocolate Cake**.

VEGAN AND GLUTEN-FREE LEMON POUND CAKE WITH LEMON-LIME GLAZE

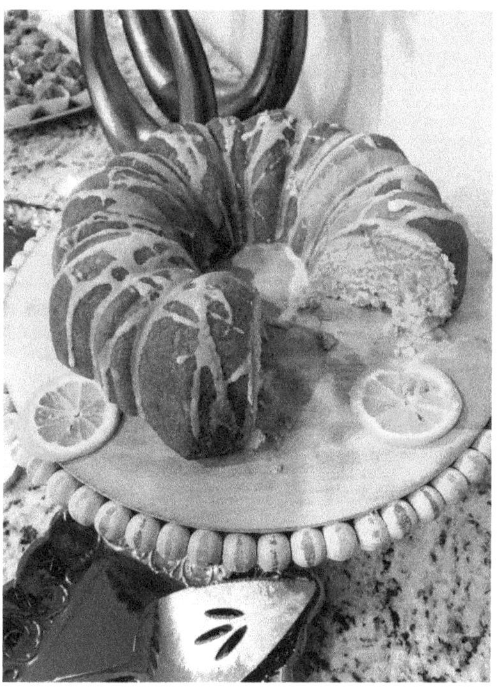

- 2 sticks plant butter, softened
- 1½ cups cane sugar
- 3½ cups gluten-free flour
- 3 teaspoons baking powder
- ¼ teaspoon ground turmeric
- ⅛ teaspoon ground green cardamom
- ¼ teaspoon salt
- 3 tablespoons chickpea aquafaba
- 1 teaspoon vanilla extract
- 1 teaspoon lemon extract
- ¼ cup fresh lemon juice
- 2 tablespoons lemon zest
- 1¼ cups almond milk

Preheat the oven to 350°F. Spray a nonstick 10-inch Bundt pan with nonstick spray. Beat the butter in a stand mixer until creamy, 2–4 minutes. Add the sugar and mix until well-combined. In a separate bowl, sift the flour, baking powder, turmeric, cardamom, and salt. Whisk the aquafaba until frothy in a separate small bowl and add to the sugar and butter. Add the flavorings, lemon juice, and lemon zest to the butter and sugar. Add in the flour mixture gradually, alternating with the milk, until they are just combined. Pour or scoop the cake batter into the prepared Bundt pan. To remove any air pockets, lightly "drop" the pan on the countertop 2–3 times. Bake for 40–45 minutes or until an inserted toothpick comes out clean. Let cool in the pan for 10–15 minutes. Place a plate over the pan, then invert the pan to release the cake. Allow the cake to cool completely before glazing with the **Lemon-Lime Glaze** (see recipe). Store the cake covered at cool room temperature for 3–5 days. Keep refrigerated if the room temperature is warm.

Makes 14–16 servings.

Lemon-Lime Glaze

- 1 cup organic confectioners' sugar, sifted
- 1 teaspoon lemon zest
- 2 teaspoons lemon juice
- 1 teaspoon lime juice

Whisk all the ingredients in a bowl. The glaze should be pourable but not watery. Add more lemon or lime juice (your preference) in small increments to reach the desired consistency. Pour over the cake and enjoy!

Makes about 1 cup.

NOTES FROM THE LAB

1. Aquafaba is the liquid in a can of chickpeas or navy beans. The typical 15.5-ounce can yields about 9 tablespoons. Invest in an oven thermometer to make sure your oven temperature is correct.
2. Plant butter is softer than regular butter, so you don't need to cream it as long.
3. Turmeric is what gives this cake its beautiful yellow color. It doesn't affect the taste, and it delivers anti-inflammatory and antioxidant benefits.
4. Green cardamom adds a lovely, zesty citrus flavor, but a little bit goes a very long way. Use too much, and it takes over in a very unpleasant way. DO NOT substitute black cardamom for green cardamom in this recipe; it has a completely different taste (smoky and minty) and does not go well with this cake.

VEGAN AND GLUTEN-FREE SWEET POTATO POUND CAKE WITH MAPLE ORANGE GLAZE

I like to think of this pound cake as what the result would be if a sweet potato pie and a pound cake had a delicious, mouth-watering baby! If sweet potatoes aren't your jam, this recipe can easily be pumpkin-ized by using pumpkin instead and adding pumpkin spice and pumpkin butter. You can thank my bestie Kim for that version!

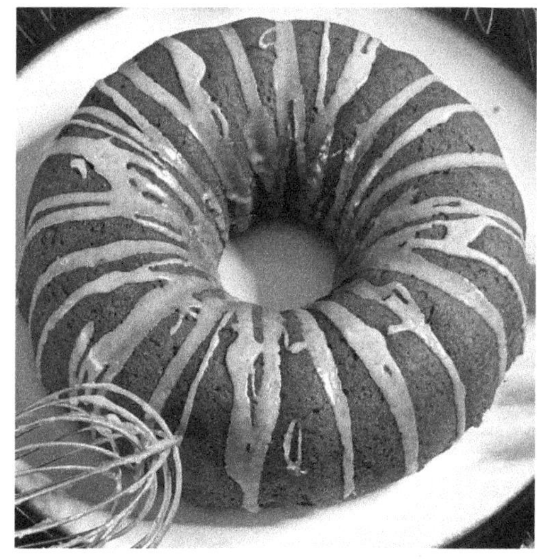

- 2 tablespoons finely ground flaxseed
- 6 tablespoons water
- 2 sticks plant butter, softened
- 1⅓ cups maple syrup
- 3 cups gluten-free flour
- 1 teaspoon nutmeg
- 2 teaspoons cinnamon
- ¼ teaspoon salt
- 2 teaspoons baking soda
- 2 cups sweet potatoes, pureed
- 2 teaspoons vanilla
- 2 tablespoons apple cider vinegar

NOTES FROM THE LAB

Make your own finely ground flaxseed: place ground flaxseed in a spice grinder and process until finely ground. If you do not have a spice grinder, a coffee grinder, pepper mill, or mortar and pestle will work as well.

Preheat the oven to 350°F. Spray a nonstick 10-inch Bundt pan with nonstick spray. Make 2 fleggs: Mix the flaxseed and water until combined and refrigerate for 10–15 minutes. The mixture should have an egg yolk-like consistency. Cream the butter and maple syrup together for 3–5 minutes in a stand mixer. Sift together the flour, nutmeg, cinnamon, salt, and baking soda in a separate bowl. Add the pureed sweet potatoes and vanilla to the butter and maple syrup mixture. Beat until well-blended. Add the apple cider vinegar and blend in. Add the fleggs and beat until well-incorporated. Add the flour mixture and beat until just combined. Do not overmix the batter. Pour into the cake pan. Lightly drop the pan on the counter 2–3 times to get rid of any air pockets. Bake for 45–50 minutes or until a toothpick inserted comes out clean. Remove from the oven and let cool in the pan for 10 minutes. Place a plate over the pan and invert the pan to release the cake. Let cool completely and then drizzle the **Maple Orange Glaze** (see recipe) over it. Store the cake covered at cool room temperature for 3–5 days. Keep refrigerated if the room temperature is warm.

Makes 14–16 servings.

NOTES FROM THE LAB

A flegg is a combination of ground flaxseed and water. To prepare, mix 2 tablespoons of ground flaxseed with 6 tablespoons of water. Place in the refrigerator while you are gathering your other ingredients. Whisk it a couple of times and the consistency should be thick like an egg yolk.

Maple Orange Glaze

- 1 cup organic confectioners' sugar
- ¼ teaspoon ground cinnamon
- ⅛ teaspoon ground nutmeg
- ¼ teaspoon vanilla extract
- 1 tablespoon maple syrup
- 1 tablespoon orange juice
- 1 tablespoon water, more to desired consistency

Sift the first 3 ingredients in a bowl. Add the next 4 ingredients and whisk together. The glaze should be thick and somewhat pourable, but not runny. Pour over the cooled **Vegan and Gluten-Free Sweet Potato Pound Cake** and enjoy! This glaze works well on cookies, too.

VEGAN BLONDIES

- 1 (15.5-ounce) can navy or Great Northern beans, rinsed (save the liquid; you will use it)
- ¾ stick plant butter
- 1 cup dark brown sugar
- ¼ cup aquafaba (the liquid in a can of beans)
- 2 tablespoons vanilla, to taste
- ½ cup pecans, pieces (toasted if desired), plus more for topping if desired)
- 1 cup whole wheat flour
- 1 teaspoon baking powder
- ½ teaspoon salt

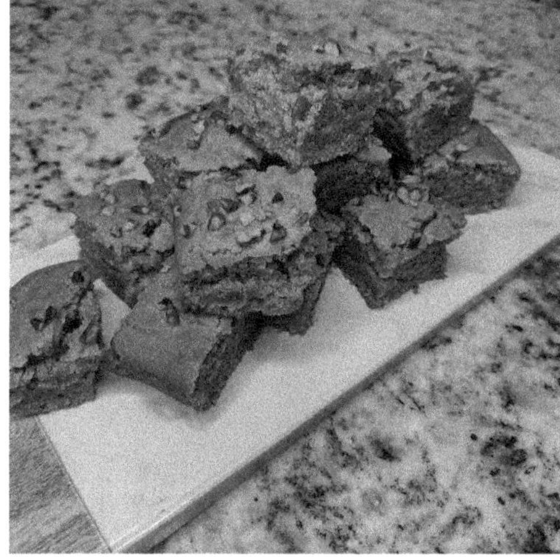

NOTES FROM THE LAB

You can also add butterscotch morsels but remember that they may not be vegan if they are made with milk.

Preheat the oven to 350°F. Line an 8 x 8-inch baking dish with parchment paper, letting it hang just over the edges. Spray with nonstick spray. Add the drained and rinsed beans to a food processor and process until smooth and creamy. (It's okay if there are a few small pieces of beans.) Melt the butter in a small saucepan over low-medium heat. Once melted, remove from the heat and stir in the sugar until combined. In a small bowl, whisk the aquafaba until slightly frothy. In a large mixing bowl, add the processed beans, vanilla, pecans, and sugar and butter mixture and stir until combined. Sift flour, baking powder, and salt into the same bowl. Stir until combined. Add in the dry ingredients. Add the aquafaba and stir until just combined. Pour into the baking dish and spread evenly, including the corners. Top with more pecans if desired. Bake for 45–50 minutes, until a toothpick inserted comes out almost dry. Allow to cool for 15–20 minutes as the blondies continue to firm up. Remove from baking dish and place on cutting board. Cut into squares and enjoy!

Makes 10–12 servings.

NOTES FROM THE LAB

Fresh Fruit Ideas

Seasonal fresh fruit makes a nice dessert. You can serve it by itself or try any of these options:

- Top fresh fruit with vanilla-flavored soy yogurt.
- Make a deconstructed apple cobbler: Chop 3–4 Granny Smith or Golden Delicious apples into evenly sized large cubes. Spray a small baking dish with nonstick spray. Add the apples in an even layer. Squeeze the juice of a lemon over them, then drizzle with 1 tablespoon of melted plant butter and 1 teaspoon of maple syrup. Sprinkle with 1–2 teaspoons light brown sugar, ¼ teaspoon salt, and 1 tablespoon cinnamon over the mixture. Cover with foil and bake at 350°F for 30 minutes. Remove the foil and increase the oven temperature to 400°F. Baste the apples with rendered apple juices and return to the oven. Bake the apples for 15 minutes. The apples should be moist and tender (like apple pie filling). Sprinkle with toasted pecans for crunch and enjoy!
- Try the above recipe with pears, peaches, or blueberries. You can also experiment with different types of nuts and spices. Adjust the oven temperature and cooking time as needed.
- Grilling fruit caramelizes the natural sugars. Lightly baste fresh pineapple or watermelon slices with sunflower or avocado oil. Grill for 3–5 minutes on each side. Your grilled fruit can be served warm or cold.

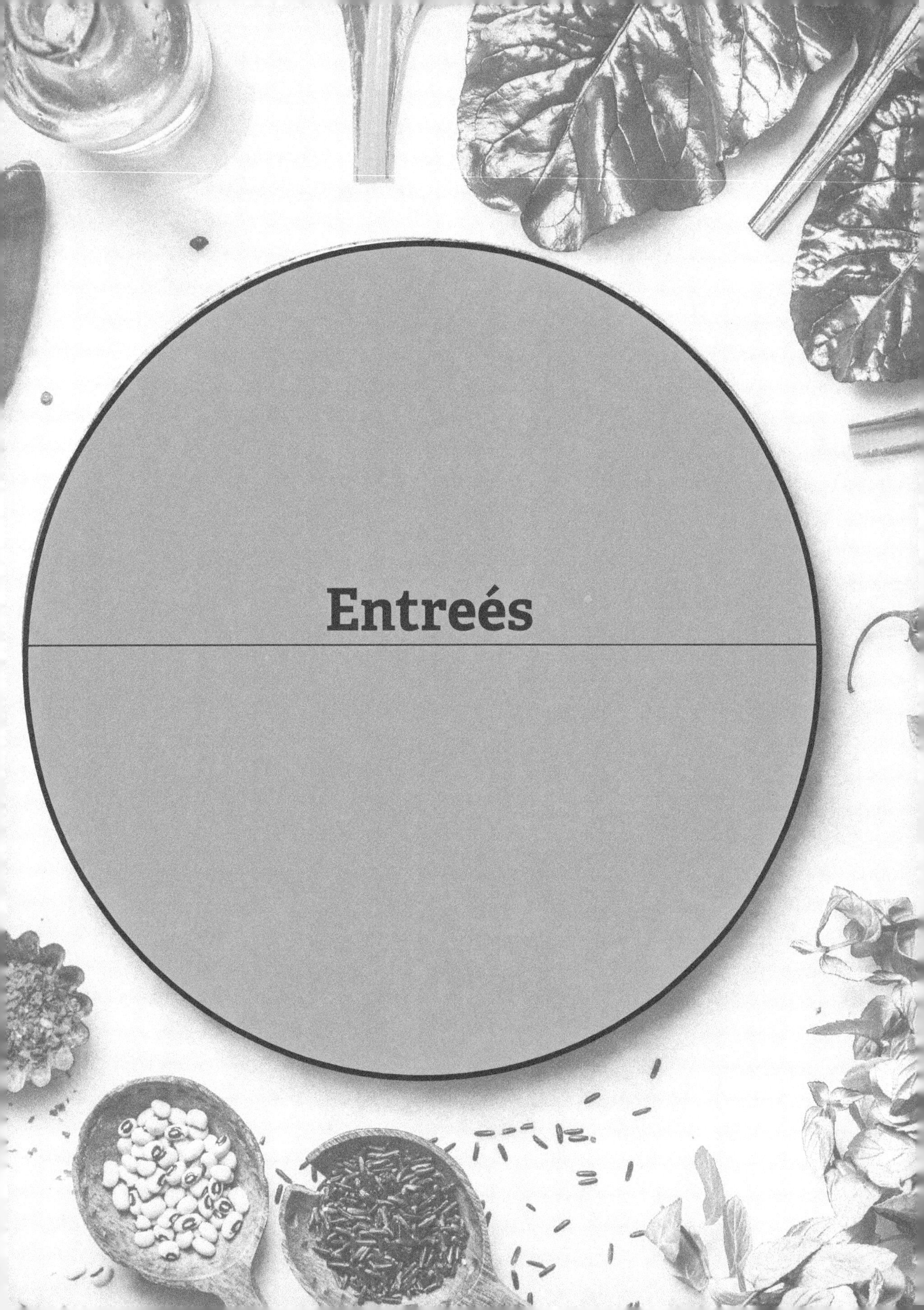

Entreés

Try these for new takes on old classics or as an introduction to something new.

AVOCADO MELT WITH BASIL AND ARUGULA PESTO

- 2 ciabatta rolls (or a crusty bread of your choice)
- Basil pesto (see recipe below)
- 2 ripe avocados, sliced
- ½ cup arugula
- 1 large beefsteak tomato, sliced

Preheat a panini press on medium heat. Slice the ciabatta bread in half horizontally. Spread the basil pesto on both sides. Place 4–6 slices of avocado on one side of the roll. Place a few sprigs of arugula on top of the avocado. Top with 1–2 large slices of tomato and cover with the other half of bread. Place the sandwich in the heated panini press and close the cover slowly so that the filling does not get squished out of the bread. Let the sandwich toast for a few minutes until it is warmed through and the outside is a nice golden color.

Makes 2 servings.

Fresh Basil Pesto

- 2 cups basil leaves, roughly chopped
- ¼ cup pine nuts
- 2–3 garlic cloves, chopped
- ½ cup grated vegan Parmesan cheese
- 1–2 cups extra virgin olive oil
- Kosher salt and pepper to taste

Add the basil and pine nuts to a food processor or blender and pulse a few times. Add the garlic and cheese and pulse some more. Scrape down the sides. Pour in the olive oil while the processor is running, stop the processor, and scrape down the sides. Add salt and pepper to taste. Use immediately or store in refrigerator for 2–3 days, covered with a thin drizzle of olive oil and with plastic wrapping pressed directly on top. To make **Basil and Arugula Pesto**, just add 1–2 handfuls of arugula to the pesto ingredients.

NOTES FROM THE LAB

If you don't have a panini press, you can use a cast-iron skillet on low-medium heat. Use a heavy-bottomed pot to press the sandwich down. Flip over after a few minutes.

NOTES FROM THE LAB

Use a blender if you don't have a food processor. Substitute sunflower seeds for the pine nuts if you have a nut allergy. To keep your pesto that pretty green color, blanch your basil in boiling water for 15 seconds, then shock in an ice bath for just a few seconds and drain before adding to this recipe.

VEGAN BEAN TACOS

- 1 tablespoon olive oil
- 1 yellow or red onion, diced
- 1 jalapeño pepper, chopped and seeded
- 2 garlic cloves, minced
- 1½ tablespoons cumin
- 1 teaspoon paprika
- ½ teaspoon Mexican oregano
- 1 teaspoon cayenne pepper
- 1 teaspoon chili powder
- 2 (14.5-ounce) cans black or pinto beans, rinsed, drained, and mashed
- 2 cups salsa
- 6–8 tortillas, warm and soft
- 1 ripe avocado, sliced
- Fresh cilantro, chopped
- Vegan sour cream for topping
- Vegan cheddar cheese for topping

Heat the olive oil in a medium skillet over medium heat. Add the onion and jalapeño pepper; cook until tender, about 5–7 minutes. Add the garlic and cook for 30–60 seconds until fragrant. Add the cumin, paprika, Mexican oregano, cayenne pepper, and chili powder. Stir in the mashed beans and salsa. Cover and cook over low heat for 5 minutes. Add to the warm tortillas and top with avocado, cilantro, sour cream, and cheese.

Makes 6–8 servings.

QUINOA AND MUSHROOM STUFFED PEPPERS

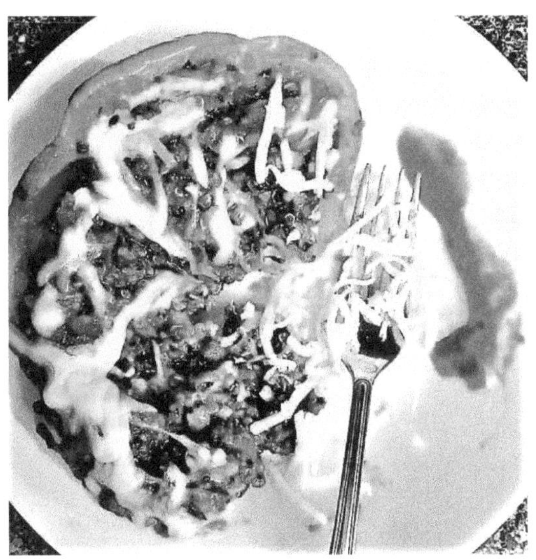

- 4 large bell peppers (red, yellow, orange)
- 1 medium yellow onion, chopped
- 1 cup baby bella mushrooms, cleaned and chopped (either by hand or a few pulses in a food processor)
- 1 teaspoon salt, divided
- 4–6 garlic cloves, minced
- 1 package plant-based ground meat
- 1 cup cooked red quinoa
- 1 (28-ounce) jar tomato sauce
- 1 cup shredded vegan mozzarella cheese

Heat the oven to 350°F. Prep the peppers by cutting the tops off and cleaning out the seeds and membranes. If the peppers cannot stand up, cut just enough off the bottoms to make a flat edge. Fill a large pot with enough water to submerge the peppers. Bring the pot to boiling over medium heat. Submerge the peppers in the boiling water and cook for about 2 minutes. Remove from the water and drain. In a large skillet, cook the onion, mushrooms, and ¼ teaspoon salt over medium heat for 5–7 minutes, stirring occasionally, until the onions are translucent and the mushrooms have released most of their liquids. Add the garlic and cook for 30–60 seconds. Add the plant-based meat and cook until warmed through. Stir in the quinoa, the rest of the salt, and 1 cup of pasta sauce; cook until warmed through. Stuff the peppers with the quinoa mixture. Stand the peppers upright in a glass baking dish. Top the peppers with the remaining pasta sauce. Cover with foil and bake for 10 minutes. Uncover and bake until the peppers are tender, about 10 more minutes. Top with cheese and serve warm. (Cheese should be just melted.)

Makes 4 servings.

SPICY VEGAN POTATO CURRY

- 4 russet potatoes, peeled and cubed
- 2 tablespoons vegetable oil
- 1 yellow onion, diced
- 2 teaspoons salt, divided
- 3 garlic cloves, minced
- 1 (1-inch) piece fresh ginger root, peeled and minced
- 2 teaspoons ground cumin
- 1½ teaspoons cayenne pepper
- 1 teaspoon curry powder
- 4 teaspoons garam masala
- 1 (14.5-ounce) can diced tomatoes
- 1 (15-ounce) can garbanzo beans (chickpeas), rinsed and drained*
- 1 (15-ounce) can green peas, drained
- 1 (14-ounce) can coconut milk

*Save the juice from the can of chickpeas to use later as an egg substitute.

Place the potatoes in a large pot and cover with salted water. Bring to a boil over high heat, then reduce heat to medium-low, cover, and simmer until just tender, about 15 minutes. Drain and allow the potatoes to steam-dry for 1 or 2 minutes with the pot covered. Meanwhile, heat the vegetable oil in a large skillet over medium heat. Add the onion and ¼ teaspoon salt and cook until it has softened and turned translucent, about 5 minutes. Add the garlic and ginger and cook for 30–60 seconds until they become fragrant. Season with cumin, cayenne pepper, curry powder, garam masala, and ½ teaspoon salt; cook for 2 more minutes. Add the tomatoes, garbanzo beans, peas, and potatoes. Pour in the coconut milk and bring to a simmer. Simmer for 5–10 minutes until the sauce is thickened and warmed through.

Makes 4–6 servings.

PHILLY CHEEZE "STEAK" SANDWICH

This recipe is a vegan take on those infamous Philly cheesesteaks I used to eat when I attended medical school at Temple University in Philadelphia. Mushrooms are an excellent meat substitute and can be grilled, baked, roasted, or sautéed.

- 2–3 tablespoons extra virgin olive oil
- 2 portobello mushroom caps, gills removed, and sliced into parallel strips about ½-inch thick
- 1 large or 2 small onions, thinly sliced
- 1 red or green bell pepper, sliced
- Kosher salt, pinch
- Black pepper, freshly ground, 2–3 grinds from a mill
- ½ teaspoon dried oregano
- ¼ teaspoon dried rosemary
- ¼ teaspoon dried thyme
- 3–4 garlic cloves, minced
- 3–4 slices vegan provolone cheese
- 2 (6-inch) whole wheat hoagie rolls, toasted

Using a cast-iron skillet or nonstick pan, swirl olive oil around the bottom 2–3 times, enough to coat the bottom. Warm over medium heat. Sauté the mushrooms, onions, and peppers for 4–7 minutes to your desired consistency. Season with salt, pepper, and herbs. Add the garlic and cook for up to a minute, until the garlic becomes fragrant. Move the pepper, mushroom, and onion mix to one side of the skillet. Cover with the cheese slices and heat until the cheese is just melted. Lift out of the skillet with a spatula, add to the rolls, and enjoy!

Makes 2 servings.

NOTES FROM THE LAB

You may substitute the oregano, thyme, and rosemary with 1½ teaspoons of Herbes de Provence.

Another way to melt the cheese is to layer the cheese over the warm filling, add to a hoagie roll, and then wrap in foil for a few minutes to melt the cheese. When you unwrap the hoagie, it's ooey-gooey goodness! This is great to reheat in the oven as well. I do not recommend microwaving the cheesesteak. Use a panini press or grill pan to get beautiful grill marks. If you're using a grill pan or stovetop grill, place a pot lid on top of the sandwich to trap the heat and make the cheese melt faster.

JERK TOFU

- 1 package extra-firm tofu, drained and dry
- ⅓ cup olive oil
- 2 tablespoons light brown sugar
- ½ tablespoon ground thyme
- 2 teaspoons ground allspice (Jamaican preferred)
- 2 teaspoons smoked paprika
- 1 teaspoon cinnamon
- ¼ teaspoon ground black pepper
- 1 teaspoon cayenne pepper
- 1 teaspoon ground cloves
- ½–1 teaspoon kosher salt

NOTES FROM THE LAB

The longer you press your tofu, the drier and firmer it will get. I recommend pressing at least overnight, so start prepping for this dish the night before.

Preheat the oven or an air fryer to 425°F. Add all the ingredients except the tofu to a mixing bowl and stir until combined. Slice the tofu into ½-inch slices. While the oven is heating, rub the spice mix liberally on all surfaces of the tofu slices and marinate for 15–20 minutes. If using an air fryer, remove the basket and spray with nonstick spray while the air fryer heats up. Bake the tofu in the oven or air fryer for 5–8 minutes, then turn over and bake another 5–8 minutes until it reaches the desired firmness. Remove from the air fryer or oven and let rest for 5 minutes before serving. The slices should be slightly dry and crispy on the outside and chewy on the inside.

Makes 2–4 servings.

PULLED "PORK" WITH HOMEMADE BBQ SAUCE

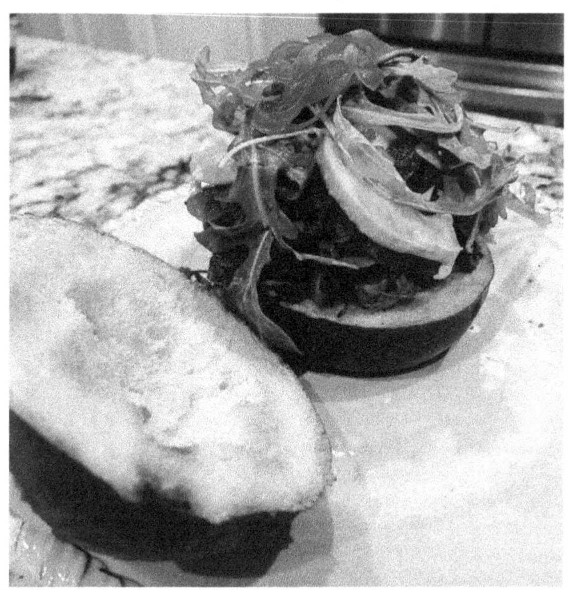

- 2 (14-ounce) cans jackfruit, drained
- 2 tablespoons olive oil
- ½ yellow onion, chopped
- 3–4 garlic cloves, minced
- ½ teaspoon chili powder
- ½ teaspoon smoked paprika
- ¼ cup tomato paste (no salt added)
- ¼ cup apple cider vinegar
- ¼ cup maple syrup
- 1 teaspoon spicy brown mustard
- ¼ teaspoon salt
- ¼ cup water, added gradually

Drain the cans of jackfruit in a large colander and rinse them under running water. Pulse the jackfruit in a food processor, or use two forks or your fingers, until it looks like pulled pork. Heat 1 tablespoon olive oil in a large skillet over medium heat. Sauté the jackfruit until desired texture, about 5–7 minutes. Remove from the skillet and place in a bowl. Add the other tablespoon of olive oil and sauté the onions until they start to soften, about 5 minutes. Add in the garlic, chili powder, and paprika, and sauté again for 30–60 seconds. Add in the tomato paste, vinegar, maple syrup, mustard, and salt, and stir well to combine. Add some water at this point to help the sauce come together and prevent it from sticking to the pan. Add water until you reach your desired consistency. Add in the jackfruit and stir well until all pieces are coated with BBQ sauce. Warm until heated through. Adjust seasoning as needed. Serve on a toasted bun with your favorite coleslaw. This pairs well with my **Vegan Southern Baked Beans**. Leftovers can be stored in an airtight container in the refrigerator for up to 1 week.

Makes 4 servings.

16-BEAN MEDLEY WITH PLANT-BASED SAUSAGE AND PURPLE RICE

This recipe is extra special to me because it was the first time I faced my fears and cooked dried beans! I simply used my mom's Power Quick Pot to avoid having to soak the beans in order to shorten the cooking time, and I was pleasantly surprised at how well everything came together! Purple rice is my new favorite rice since it is more flavorful and healthier than white rice and adds a nice texture to the dish. I used some homemade veggie stock seasoned with chicken-flavored seasoning for even more flavor! Be aware that if you do not soak your beans first, then you will need to run them through a second cycle of your MultiPot.

- 2–3 tablespoons extra virgin olive oil
- 1 yellow onion, chopped
- 1 package plant-based chicken-style Italian sausage, removed from the casing and cubed
- 6–8 garlic cloves, minced
- ½ of a 16-ounce bag of bean soup mix, sorted and rinsed
- 4–6 cups of vegan chicken stock or vegetable stock
- 1 teaspoon cumin
- 1 teaspoon ground white pepper
- ½ teaspoon smoked paprika
- 1 teaspoon garlic powder
- 1 teaspoon onion powder
- 1 cup purple rice
- Cilantro, chopped, for garnish (optional)

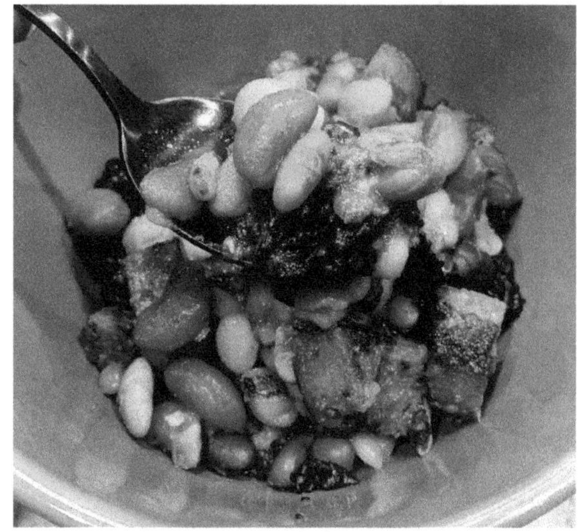

Add olive oil to a MultiPot and sauté the onion and sausage until they are browned, 5–6 minutes. Add the garlic and sauté for 30–60 seconds, until you can just start to smell the garlic. Remove the sausage mix from the pot. Place the beans in the MultiPot and add the stock. Add the cumin, white pepper, smoked paprika, garlic powder, and onion powder, and stir. Cover with the lid and cook using the "beans" setting of the pressure cooking function. When the cooking cycle is done, check the beans for doneness. The beans should be plump and just give when pressed with a fork. If they are not, then cook them for another cycle. While the beans are cooking, cook the purple rice according to its package instructions. Once the beans are cooked, remove the lid and add the onion, sausage, and garlic mixture and stir until combined. Serve warm over the cooked purple rice. Top with cilantro if desired.

If you do not have a MultiPot, use a nonstick skillet to sauté the onion, sausage, and garlic over medium heat as stated above, cook the beans according to the package directions, and then just combine everything or serve the sausage and bean mix over the rice.

Makes 6–8 servings.

CAULIFLOWER RICE STIR-FRY WITH DUCK SAUCE AND HOT MUSTARD

Stir-Fry

- 3–4 tablespoons garlic stir-fry oil
- 4 ounces baby bella mushrooms, cut into strips
- ½ red onion, cut into strips
- 1 red bell pepper, cut into strips
- 1-inch knob fresh ginger, grated and divided
- 4 garlic cloves, minced and divided
- ¼–½ block extra-firm tofu, drained of liquid and roughly chopped
- ¼ teaspoon ground turmeric
- ½ cauliflower head, riced (you may use frozen or make your own with a food processor or blender)
- ¼–½ cup soy sauce (you may also use tamari or coconut aminos)
- 1 cup bean sprouts, rinsed
- 1 cup frozen green peas

Add 1–2 tablespoons of oil to a wok over medium heat. Add the mushrooms, onion, and bell pepper to the wok, stirring frequently, and cook for 3–4 minutes. Add half the garlic and half of the ginger and cook for 30–60 seconds, until fragrant. In a separate small skillet, add 1 tablespoon of stir-fry oil over medium heat. Add the tofu and turmeric. Break the tofu apart with a fork and "scramble" until it looks like a scrambled egg, about 3–5 minutes. Add the cauliflower rice and the remainder of the garlic and ginger to the wok and cook for another 3 minutes. Add the soy sauce and stir. Add the bean sprouts and peas. Stir until well-blended and warm throughout. Add more sauce to taste. Serve the stir-fry with duck sauce and hot mustard. Store any unused portion covered in the refrigerator for 2–3 days.

Makes 6 servings.

Hot Mustard

- 1 teaspoon yellow mustard
- 2 tablespoons ground mustard powder
- 2 tablespoons rice wine vinegar
- 1 teaspoon honey
- ½ teaspoon water
- ¼ teaspoon ground ginger

Combine all ingredients to a bowl and whisk until smooth. Add more water as needed to reach desired consistency and thickness.

Makes ¼ cup.

Duck Sauce

- 3–4 tablespoons apricot jam
- 1½ tablespoons rice wine vinegar
- ¼ teaspoon ground mustard
- ¼ teaspoon garlic powder
- ⅛ teaspoon ginger powder (fresh is better if you have it on hand)

Mash the apricot jam with a fork to break down any large pieces of fruit. Add the remaining ingredients and whisk until blended well.

Makes ¼ cup.

VEGAN LENTIL, KALE, AND SAUSAGE PASTA

- 2½ cups no-sodium vegetable broth
- ¾ cup dry brown lentils
- 1 teaspoon salt, divided
- 1 bay leaf
- ¼ cup olive oil
- 1 large onion, chopped
- 1 teaspoon dried thyme
- 1 teaspoon dried oregano
- 1 teaspoon salt
- ½ teaspoon black pepper
- 8 ounces vegan sausage, cut into ¼-inch slices
- 1 bunch of kale, stems removed and leaves coarsely chopped
- 1 (12-ounce) package whole wheat rotini pasta
- 2 tablespoons nutritional yeast (optional)

Bring the vegetable broth, lentils, ½ teaspoon of salt, and bay leaf to a boil in a saucepan over high heat. Reduce the heat to medium-low, cover, and simmer until the lentils are tender, about 20 minutes. Do not boil. Add additional broth if needed to keep the lentils moist. Discard the bay leaf once done. As the lentils simmer, heat the olive oil in a skillet over medium-high heat. Add the onion, thyme, oregano, ½ teaspoon salt, and pepper. Cook and stir for 1 minute, then add the sausage. Reduce the heat to medium-low, and cook until the onion has softened, about 5–7 minutes. Meanwhile, bring a large pot of lightly salted water to a boil over high heat. Add the kale and rotini pasta. Cook until the rotini is *al dente,* about 8 minutes. Remove ½ cup of the cooking water and set it aside. Drain the pasta and kale, then return them to the pot and stir in the lentils and onion and sausage mixture. Use the reserved cooking liquid to adjust the moisture of the dish to your liking. Sprinkle with nutritional yeast and serve.

Makes 6 servings.

RED RICE, BROWN LENTIL, AND MUSHROOM BURGER

- 2 tablespoons ground flaxseed
- 6 tablespoons water
- 2–3 tablespoons extra virgin olive oil
- 1 cup baby bella mushrooms, chopped
- 1 cup brown lentils, cooked according to package instructions
- 1 cup red rice, cooked according to package instructions
- 3 tablespoons liquid smoke
- ¼ cup Worcestershire sauce (vegan preferred)
- 3 teaspoons onion powder
- 3 teaspoons garlic powder
- 3 teaspoons dried oregano
- ½ teaspoon dried thyme
- 2–3 teaspoons smoked paprika
- 1 cup panko bread crumbs

NOTES FROM THE LAB

If you are serving these on hamburger buns, be sure to make your patties the same size as the bun. Unlike meat patties, these babies don't shrink, so what you make is what you get!

Make 2 fleggs: combine the flaxseed and water. Whisk together and place in the refrigerator for 10 minutes. Warm olive oil in a large pan over medium heat. Add mushrooms and sauté until they release their liquid and soften, about 3–5 minutes. Allow to cool slightly. Combine the mushrooms and all the remaining ingredients, including the fleggs, in a large bowl. Form into patties. Refrigerate for 30 minutes. While waiting for the patties to set, prep your grill. Wipe down the grates with olive oil and preheat over medium heat. Remove the patties from the refrigerator and place them onto the preheated grill. Cook for 3–4 minutes on one side, then turn over and cook for another 3–4 minutes. Remove from the grill and allow to "rest" before serving. Serve on toasted buns with your favorite condiments.

TOFU PARMIGIANA

- 2 tablespoons olive oil
- 2 packages extra-firm tofu, drained and pressed, cut into ½-inch-thick slices
- 1 (24-ounce) jar tomato basil garlic tomato sauce (I prefer Prego)
- 2 teaspoons ground fennel
- 2 teaspoons garlic powder
- 1 teaspoon onion powder
- 16 ounces shredded vegan mozzarella cheese
- 4 ounces vegan Parmesan cheese, grated
- Salt to taste

Preheat the oven to 350°F. Spray a baking dish with nonstick spray. In a skillet over medium heat, heat oil and place tofu in the skillet. Sear each side until golden brown on all sides. While the tofu sears, pour the tomato sauce in a bowl and add the fennel, onion, and garlic powder. Stir until combined. Lay half of the browned tofu in a single layer in a baking dish. Top with the spaghetti sauce and mozzarella cheese. Top with another layer of browned tofu, sauce, and cheese. Top with Parmesan cheese. Cover the dish with aluminum foil. Bake at 350°F for 30 minutes. Allow to cool for 5 minutes and serve warm.

Makes 4 servings.

VEGAN "BUTTER CHICKEN"

Surprise! This restaurant-quality dish contains neither butter nor chicken. For added creaminess you can certainly add butter, but to keep it vegan, use plant butter. This is my version of the classic recipe that celebrates many Indian spices such as garam masala, which is a fantastic combination of many of the "C" spices: cloves, cumin, coriander, cardamom, and cinnamon, as well as black pepper and nutmeg. I made a version of garam masala that uses cinnamon, cardamom, and cloves for this recipe, but you can also buy it ready-made. If you do, adjust the remaining ingredients based on what your mixture contains.

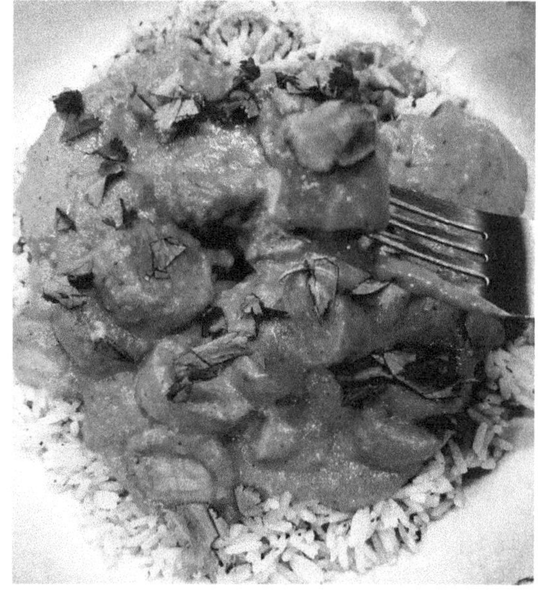

Marinade

- ¼ cup vegan yogurt
- 1 tablespoon garlic, minced
- ½ tablespoon ginger, minced
- 2 teaspoons garam masala
- ½ teaspoon ground turmeric
- 1 teaspoon ground cumin
- ½ teaspoon chili powder
- ½ teaspoon salt

Butter Sauce

- 2 tablespoons olive oil
- ½ large onion or 1 medium onion, diced
- ½ tablespoon grated ginger
- 1 tablespoon minced garlic
- ½ teaspoon ground coriander
- ¾ teaspoon ground cumin
- ¾ teaspoon garam masala
- 1 (14-ounce) can crushed tomatoes
- 1 teaspoon chili powder
- ½ teaspoon salt
- 1–2 tablespoons water
- ½ cup full-fat coconut milk
- ½ tablespoon sugar
- ½ teaspoon dried fenugreek leaves
- 12–16 ounces king mushrooms, prepped (see below)
- ¼ cup cilantro, chopped, for garnish

King Oyster Mushrooms

- 1–2 pounds king oyster mushrooms
- 2 tablespoons neutral oil (avocado or olive oil)
- Kosher salt, pinch
- ½ teaspoon black pepper
- 1 teaspoon cumin

Prep the mushrooms: Clean the mushrooms with a damp cloth or by rinsing them under running water and then patting dry. Cut the tops of the mushrooms off (these can be used as scallop substitutes in another recipe), leaving just the cylinder-shaped stems. Slice the stems into round disks about ½-inch-thick. Cut diagonal hash marks on one side of each mushroom piece. Add 2 tablespoons of avocado or olive oil to a skillet over medium-high heat. Once the skillet is hot, add in a pinch of kosher salt, ½ teaspoon of black pepper, 1 teaspoon cumin, and stir into the warm oil. Add the mushrooms and sauté for about 2–3 minutes on each side. Remove from the heat.

In a bowl, combine the king oyster mushrooms with all of the marinade ingredients. Marinate for at least 30 minutes in the refrigerator. Remove from the refrigerator. Heat oil in a skillet over medium heat. Add the onions to the skillet and cook until they are translucent and soft, about 5 minutes. Add the garlic and ginger and sauté for 30–60 seconds, stirring frequently. Add in the coriander, cumin, and garam masala and cook for 20–30 seconds until fragrant, stirring constantly. Add the crushed tomatoes, chili powder, and salt. Simmer for 10–15 minutes until the sauce thickens. Remove from the heat. Place the mixture in a blender and puree until smooth. Add a couple of tablespoons of water to help loosen it up if needed. Place the puree back into the skillet and add the coconut milk, sugar, and fenugreek leaves. Rub or crush the leaves between your fingers before adding them to the sauce to release more flavor. Add the king oyster mushrooms to the sauce and sauté for 5 minutes until warmed through. Garnish with chopped cilantro and serve over basmati or jasmine rice.

Makes 6 servings.

BBQ RIBZ

- 1 pound of sliced seitan
- 1 tablespoon onion powder
- 1 tablespoon garlic powder
- ¼ teaspoon ground black pepper
- ¼ teaspoon kosher salt
- 4 tablespoons extra virgin olive oil
- 1 cup **Tablespoon BBQ Sauce** (see recipe)

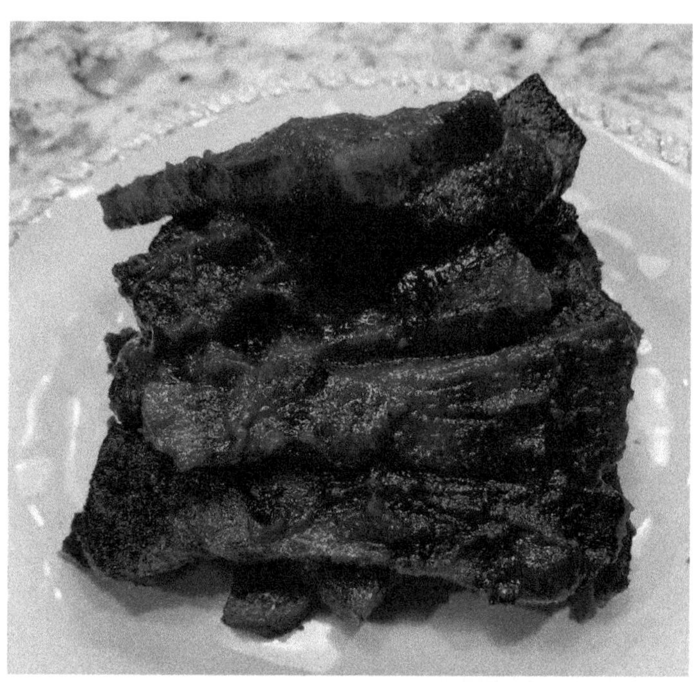

Season the seitan with the onion powder, garlic powder, salt, and pepper. Stack the seitan slices in a neat pile and cut them into ½-inch-wide strips. Heat a grill pan over medium heat and add 2 tablespoons of olive oil. Add the strips of seitan and cook for 3–4 minutes on one side; then turn and cook on the other side for another 2–3 minutes. Add more olive oil if the pieces start to stick to the pan. Once both sides have beautiful grill marks, remove from the heat and slather with **Tablespoon BBQ Sauce**. Serve while warm.

NOTES FROM THE LAB

You can season and marinate your seitan however you like before grilling. If you don't have a grill pan, you can use a nonstick skillet instead.

Tablespoon BBQ sauce

- 1 (6-ounce) can tomato paste
- 1 tablespoon onion powder
- 1 tablespoon garlic powder
- 1 tablespoon chili powder
- 1 tablespoon smoked paprika
- 1 tablespoon liquid smoke
- 1 tablespoon coconut aminos
- ¼ cup apple cider vinegar
- ½ cup maple syrup
- 1 tablespoon spicy brown mustard
- ½ teaspoon salt
- ¼ teaspoon ground black pepper
- 1 ounce dark chocolate or 1 square of a 3.5-ounce bar
- ½ cup–1 cup water, to desired consistency

Place all ingredients (except for the dark chocolate) with ½ cup water in a wide sauté pan or frying pan and warm over medium heat, stirring frequently. Simmer until the ingredients are well-blended, about 5–7 minutes. DO NOT BOIL. Add more water to reach the desired consistency. Add dark chocolate and stir until melted.

NOTES FROM THE LAB

If you want more heat, add several dashes of hot sauce or ⅛ teaspoon cayenne pepper. For smokier flavor, add more smoked paprika or liquid smoke. Add an extra splash of maple syrup if you prefer sweeter barbecue sauce. You can also add more vinegar too. FYI: Liquid aminos is a gluten-free, low-sodium option that can be used in place of Worcestershire sauce in recipes.

"CRAB" CAKES

- 2 tablespoons ground flaxseed
- 6 tablespoons water
- 1 (20-ounce) can jackfruit, rinsed and drained
- 1–2 cups vegetable oil of choice, divided (use one with a high smoke point, such as grapeseed, avocado, or sunflower oil)
- ⅓ cup red onion, chopped
- 3–4 garlic cloves, minced
- 1¼ cups whole wheat panko bread crumbs
- ¼ cup fresh dill, chopped
- 1 teaspoon onion powder
- 1 teaspoon garlic powder
- ½ tablespoon Old Bay Seasoning
- ¼ teaspoon salt
- ½ teaspoon cayenne powder
- ¼ teaspoon smoked paprika
- 2–3 tablespoons vegan fish sauce or vegetable broth

Make 2 fleggs: Mix flaxseed and water until combined and refrigerate for 10–15 minutes. The mixture should have an egg yolk-like consistency. Pulse the jackfruit in a food processor until it looks like lump crabmeat (3–4 pulses). Add to a large mixing bowl. Add 1–2 tablespoons of oil to large skillet. Sauté the onion over medium heat until translucent, about 5 minutes. Add the garlic and sauté for 30–60 seconds or until it becomes fragrant. Remove from the heat and allow to cool for a few minutes, then add the onion and garlic mix to the bowl with jackfruit. Add the remaining ingredients except for the remaining oil. Heat the rest of the oil in a large cast-iron skillet over medium heat. While the oil is warming, scoop out the jackfruit using a ¼ cup measuring scoop. Form into patties. Cook on each side for 4–5 minutes until crispy and golden brown. Serve warm.

Makes 4 servings.

SOUTHWESTERN BOWL

This is my version of my favorite dish at Tacos 4 Life. The fresh flavors and different textures feel like a party in my mouth!

- ½ cup chicken alternative, chopped
- 1 cup rice of choice, cooked according to package directions
- ½ cup diced tomatoes, drained (save the juice for the dressing below)
- ½ cup black beans, rinsed and cooked
- ⅓ cup frozen corn, thawed and cooked
- 1 ripe avocado, sliced
- ½ cup fresh cilantro, chopped, for garnish
- Tortilla strips for topping
- Vegan sour cream for topping
- Vegan cheddar cheese for topping

Prepare the chicken substitute or your protein of choice per package instructions. Using a wide, shallow bowl, layer the bottom with cooked rice. Add a layer of chicken substitute. Lay out the next layer in quarter sections: add the tomatoes, beans, corn, and avocado. Drizzle with **Southwestern Dressing** (see below). Top with the cilantro, tortilla strips, sour cream, and cheddar as desired.

Southwestern Dressing

- Tomato juice from can that was drained above
- 2 tablespoons Greek or vegan yogurt
- 1 teaspoon lime juice or lime vinegar
- ½ teaspoon lime zest
- ⅛ teaspoon cumin
- ⅛ teaspoon chili powder
- Pinch of Mexican oregano
- ½ teaspoon fresh dill or ⅛ teaspoon dried dill
- ⅛ teaspoon smoked paprika
- ½ teaspoon garlic powder
- ½ teaspoon onion powder

Whisk together all the ingredients in a bowl and drizzle over the **Southwestern Bowl.** Store leftovers in a sealed container in the refrigerator for 2–3 days.

Makes 2 servings.

VEGAN LENTIL TACOS

Lentils make a nice substitute for the traditional beef that usually goes in tacos.

- 1 cup dried brown lentils
- 1 (6-ounce) can of tomato paste
- 2 tablespoons chili powder
- 1 teaspoon cumin
- 1 teaspoon paprika
- ½ teaspoon ground Mexican oregano or regular oregano (regular oregano will work too)
- 6 corn tortillas or taco shells
- Shredded iceberg lettuce

Optional toppings:

- Guacamole
- Pico de gallo
- Vegan sour cream
- Vegan cheddar cheese
- Cilantro
- Green onions, chopped

Place the lentils in a saucepan and add enough water to cover them by at least an inch. Heat over medium heat. Cover with a lid and bring to a boil, then reduce the heat and simmer until tender, about 20 minutes (there may still be a small amount of water in the pot). Stir in the tomato paste and spices and cook until warmed through and desired thickness. Spoon the lentil mix into the taco shells or tortillas and top with lettuce and other recommended toppings.

Makes 6 servings.

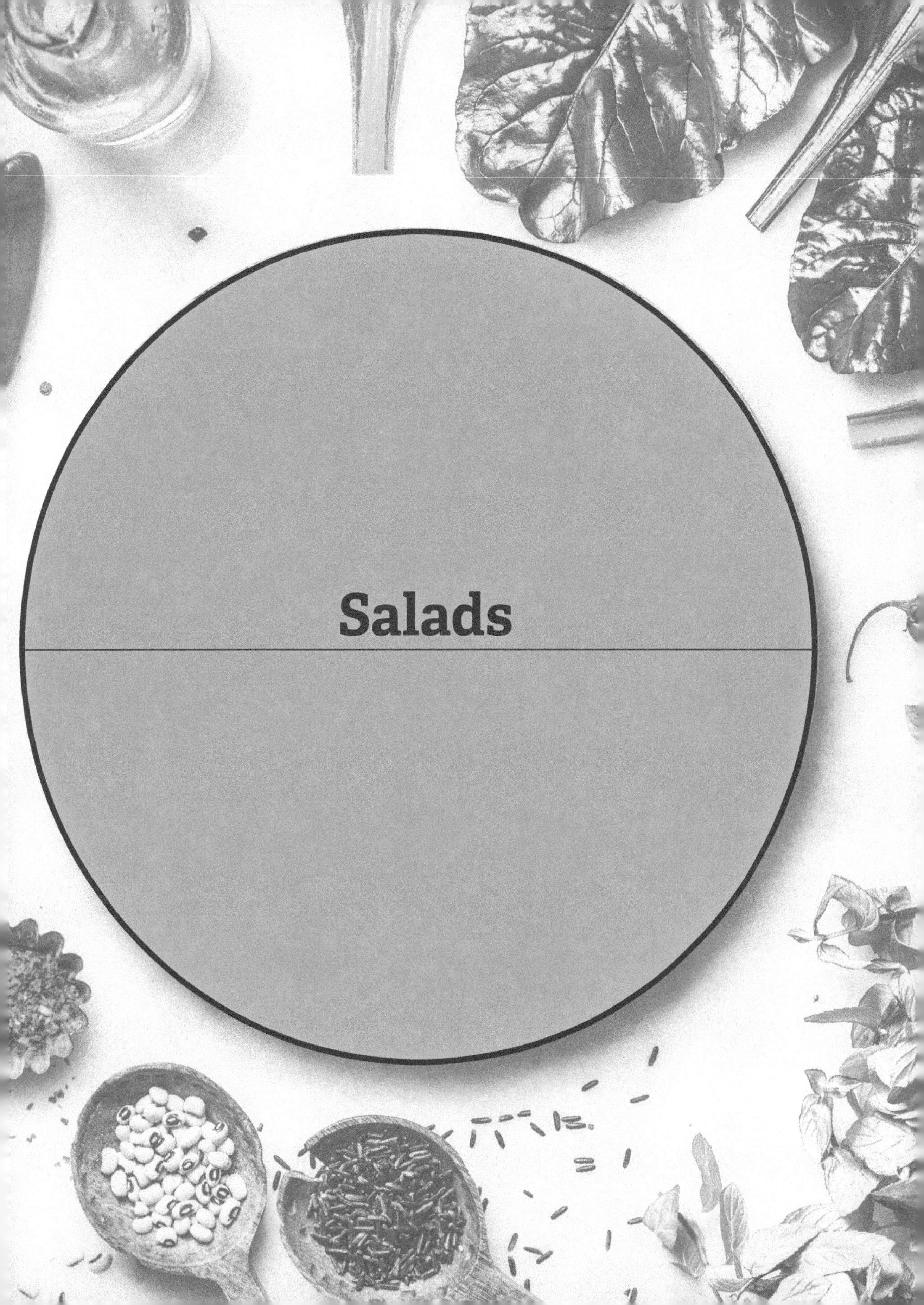

Salads

Colorful and full of nutrients, salads are a wonderful way to get some of your daily required servings of fruits, vegetables, and proteins. Remember: the more varied the ingredients, textures, and tastes, the more exciting the salad is! Salads are ideal because you can use whatever you have on hand. Keep your fridge well-stocked with produce, and you can make a healthy salad whenever you want. You can make your own vegan dressings, too. Vinaigrettes are especially easy because all they require are 1 part acid (lemon juice, wine, or vinegar) and 2–3 parts oil (olive, grapeseed, avocado, etc.). You can also add salt, pepper, fresh herbs, and spices to taste.

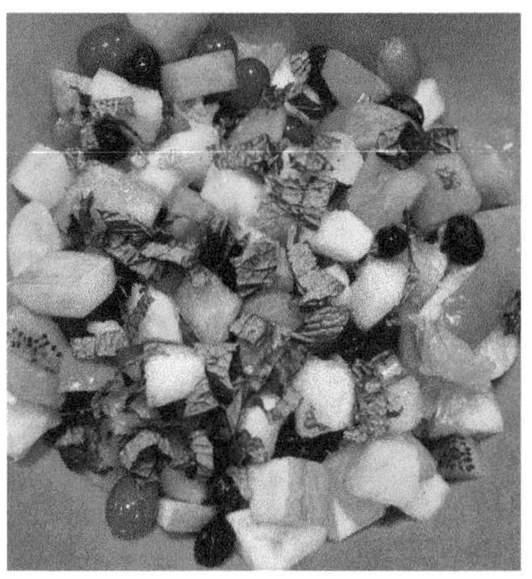

FRESH FRUIT SALAD

- 1 Fuji or Gala apple, cubed
- ½ cup pineapple, cubed
- 1 orange, peeled, sections separated and white fibrous parts removed, chopped
- 1 grapefruit or pomelo, peeled, sections separated and white fibrous parts removed, chopped
- 1–2 kiwis, cubed
- 1 cup cantaloupe or honeydew melon, cubed
- ½ cup grapes, halved
- ½ cup berries (blueberries, strawberries, or raspberries), halved
- 1 mango, cubed
- 3–4 mint leaves
- 1 tablespoon honey (optional)

Place all the fruits in a large bowl. Wash and dry the mint leaves. Chiffonade the mint leaves: Stack them in a pile and roll into a bundle lengthwise (like a cigar). Using a sharp chef's knife, chop leaves into small ribbons, starting at the top of the bundle (the shorter end). Discard the tough stems at the ends. Add the mint and honey to the fruit bowl and stir gently until items are just combined.

Serve immediately. Store any remaining fruit salad in an airtight container in the refrigerator for 3–5 days.

Makes 8 servings.

NOTES FROM THE LAB

This fruit salad is flavorful and packed full of antioxidants, vitamins, and minerals. The combination of fruits provides a nice contrast in textures and tastes. Fresh mint adds a surprising bit of freshness and color. Keep in mind: these are the fruits I like to use, but of course, you can substitute whatever you like. I also add a squeeze of honey, which can be omitted to make this vegan.

MEXICAN-INSPIRED REFRIGERATOR "CLEAN OUT"

- ½ cup corn kernels
- ½ cup black beans, rinsed and drained if using canned beans
- 1–2 celery ribs, diced
- ½ cup cilantro, chopped
- ½ green bell pepper, diced
- ½ red bell pepper, diced
- 1 small jalapeño pepper, seeded and diced
- 2 cups cherry tomatoes, halved
- ½ red onion, diced
- Juice and zest of one lime
- ¼ teaspoon ground cumin
- ¼ teaspoon chili powder
- Pinch of ground cayenne pepper
- Pinch of kosher salt (optional)
- 1 ripe avocado, sliced (optional)

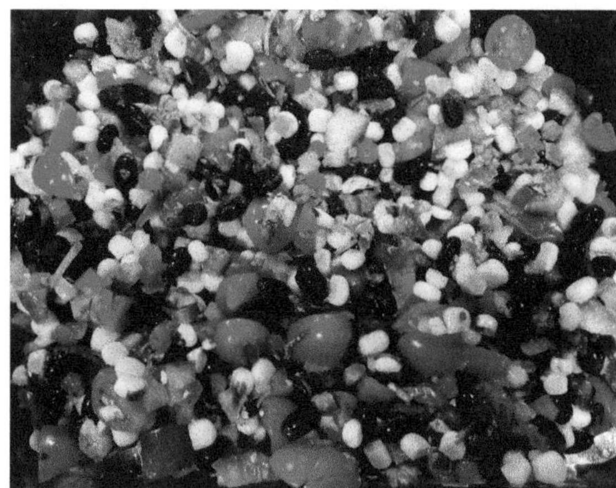

Place the corn kernels in a nonstick skillet over low-medium heat. Toast the kernels until they just start to turn brown. Allow to cool slightly. Place in a large bowl and add the remaining ingredients. Lay the avocado slices on top. Serve with tortilla chips. Refrigerate leftovers in an airtight container for 3–5 days (but trust me, it won't last that long).

Makes 4–6 servings.

SUPER SALAD

- ½–1 small red onion, thinly sliced
- 3–4 cups of greens (kale, spinach, or salad mix)
- 6–8 mini bell peppers (red, yellow, orange), sliced
- 1 cup cherry or grape tomatoes, halved
- 5–6 large brussels sprouts, prepped and thinly sliced (use a mandoline if available)
- ½ cup fresh fruit of choice (apple slices, berries, oranges)
- ¼ cup chopped nuts or sunflower seeds, toasted
- ½ cup red kidney beans, rinsed and drained
- 8 ounces grilled protein such as seitan, tofu, or tempeh
- ¼ cup vegan feta cheese (optional)
- Low-fat dressing or vinaigrette of your choice

Place the sliced onions in ice water for 5–10 minutes, then drain. While the onions are soaking, mix the greens, peppers, tomatoes, and brussels sprouts in a large bowl. Add the onions, fruit, nuts or seeds, and beans. Stir to mix. Place in serving bowls and top with protein. Top with crumbled feta cheese. Drizzle lightly with low-fat salad dressing or vinaigrette and serve immediately. Store remaining salad in an airtight container in the refrigerator for 2–3 days.

Makes 4 servings.

TRICOLOR PASTA AND RED BEAN SALAD

- 6 ounces tricolor whole wheat pasta
- 1 (15-ounce) can red kidney beans, rinsed and drained
- 1 medium red onion, diced
- 1 cup cherry tomatoes, halved
- 1 bell pepper, diced
- ½ teaspoon cumin
- Vinaigrette of your choice
- 4 ounces vegan Parmesan cheese, shaved
- ¼ cup fresh parsley, chopped

Cook pasta according to package directions. Drain the pasta. Add to a large serving bowl. Add the beans, onion, tomatoes, bell pepper, and cumin; combine well. Toss with vinaigrette. Top with shaved Parmesan cheese and parsley. Serve chilled.

Makes 6–8 servings.

VEGAN CAESAR SALAD

The Caesar salad is a classic, but the dressing is definitely not vegan-friendly. This recipe changes that! Capers provide the saltiness instead of anchovies, so no need to add extra salt.

Dressing

- 1 ripe avocado
- Juice of 1 lemon
- 2–4 garlic cloves, minced
- 1½ tablespoons capers, rinsed
- 1 tablespoon Dijon mustard
- 1–2 tablespoons water
- 1–2 teaspoons freshly ground black pepper
- 3 tablespoons extra virgin olive oil

Add all ingredients to a blender except the olive oil and puree until smooth. With the motor running, drizzle in the olive oil. Stop and scrape down the sides with a spatula. Add more water in teaspoon increments to reach your desired consistency.

Salad

- 1 head of romaine lettuce, torn or cut into large pieces
- ¼ cup vegan Parmesan cheese, shaved from a block
- 2 cups croutons

Add the romaine lettuce to a large bowl. Add the dressing and toss until the lettuce is well-coated. Top with shaved vegan Parmesan cheese and croutons. Season with freshly ground black pepper and serve.

Makes 4 servings.

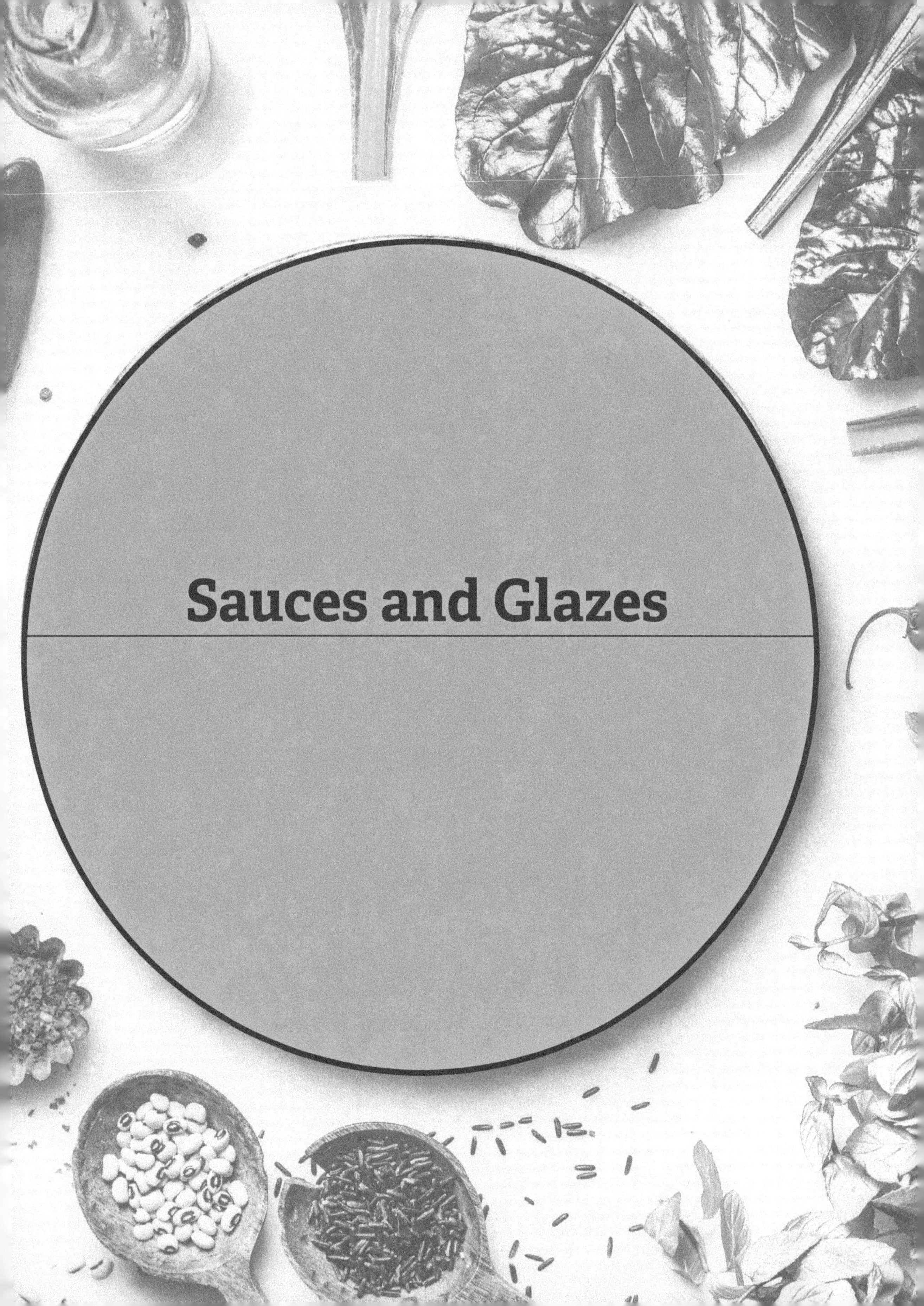

Sauces and Glazes

These add a layer of flavor, moisture, or visual appeal to any dish. Think of them as accessories: No well-dressed plate would be seen without them!

MEXICAN PESTO

This is a Mexican-inspired version of pesto that folks with nut allergies can enjoy as well! It makes a great topping for burritos or quesadillas, roasted chicken breast, grilled salmon, or sandwiches.

- ½ cup sunflower seeds
- 3–4 small garlic cloves
- 1 ripe avocado
- 3 cups fresh cilantro leaves, roughly chopped
- ½ teaspoon chili powder
- ¼ teaspoon cumin
- ¼ teaspoon salt
- 1½ cups avocado oil
- 1 cup Cotija cheese
- 1 teaspoon lime juice

Place the sunflower seeds and garlic in a food processor fitted with a metal blade. Process for 15 seconds. Add the avocado and process for 30 seconds. Next, add the cilantro, chili powder, cumin and salt. With the processor running, slowly pour avocado oil into the bowl through the feed tube and process until thoroughly pureed. Add the Cotija cheese and lime juice and puree for up to 1 minute. Use right away or store in the fridge or freezer with a thin layer of olive oil on top, covered by plastic wrap.

Makes 2 cups.

RASPBERRY SOY SAUCE GLAZE

- ¼ cup raspberry preserves
- 2 teaspoons Dijon mustard
- 2 teaspoons soy sauce (or coconut aminos)
- ¼ cup water
- 1 teaspoon ginger powder

Combine all ingredients in a small saucepan and simmer over low heat until the raspberry preserves are dissolved. Whisk until smooth. Drizzle over your chosen protein and marinate in the refrigerator for 30 minutes. Grill or bake and use any excess glaze to baste while cooking. Enjoy!

Makes ½ cup.

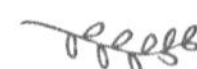

ASIAN-INSPIRED MARINADE

- 2 tablespoons sesame oil
- ¼ cup coconut aminos or low-sodium soy sauce
- ¼ cup rice vinegar
- 1 tablespoon Five-spice powder
- 1 teaspoon garlic powder
- 1 teaspoon ginger powder
- 1 tablespoon honey
- 1 teaspoon horseradish
- 1 teaspoon sesame seeds

Mix all ingredients together in a bowl and whisk together until well-blended. Use to marinate 1 pound of tofu, tempeh, seitan, or vegetables. Store any unused marinade in the refrigerator for up to 1 week in an airtight container.

Makes ½ cup.

MITCHELL AND MOM'S SPAGHETTI SAUCE

I created this recipe while showing my son how to make spaghetti one night. This is our version of the Italian classic "gravy" (meat-free, of course).

- 2 tablespoons olive oil (or plant butter)
- 1 onion, chopped
- 4 garlic cloves, pressed or finely minced
- ¼ teaspoon crushed red pepper flakes
- 1 (28-ounce) can San Marzano tomatoes, crushed (with juices)
- 2 tablespoons dried oregano
- 1 teaspoon ground fennel
- 2 tablespoons garlic powder
- 1 tablespoon onion powder
- 1 teaspoon kosher salt
- ½ teaspoon black pepper
- ½ teaspoon sugar
- 1 cup fresh basil, chopped

Heat olive oil in a large saucepan over medium heat. Add the onion and sauté for 5 minutes, stirring occasionally, until softened. Add the garlic and cook for 30–60 seconds, until it becomes fragrant. Add all other ingredients except for the fresh basil and bring to a boil. Reduce heat to low, cover, and simmer for 20–25 minutes, keeping a close eye on it, until the sauce has thickened. Use a wooden spoon to break up the tomatoes as the sauce continues to heat. If you prefer a smoother sauce, you can also puree it with an immersion blender (after you remove from heat) until it reaches your desired consistency. Remove from the heat and stir in the fresh basil before serving over cooked pasta.

Makes 2 cups.

DARK CHOCOLATE BALSAMIC GLAZE

- ⅓ cup dark chocolate balsamic vinegar
- 2/3 cup extra virgin olive oil
- 2 teaspoons Dijon mustard
- 2 teaspoons maple syrup
- ½ teaspoon salt

Add all ingredients to a bottle or jar with a secure top and shake until well-blended. Store in the refrigerator for 1–2 weeks. Shake well before each use.

Makes 1½ cups.

VEGAN ALFREDO SAUCE

- 1 stick plant butter
- 1½ cups soy or almond milk
- 1 tablespoon whole wheat flour
- ¼ teaspoon nutmeg
- 5–6 garlic cloves, minced
- 2 cups vegan Parmesan cheese, shredded

Add the butter and milk to a large skillet. Simmer over low heat for 2 minutes. Whisk in the flour and nutmeg and cook for 1 minute. Add the garlic and cook for 30–60 seconds, until the garlic is fragrant. Whisk in the Parmesan cheese until melted. Add to a cooked pasta of your choice and serve immediately.

Makes 2–3 cups.

VEGAN GREEN GODDESS DRESSING

This recipe has a lot of ingredients, but trust me, it is worth it! This was a collaboration between my mom and me. She wanted to use watercress and I prefer arugula, so I have included both for you to decide which delicious option you prefer.

- ¼ cup apple cider vinegar
- 1 cup basil
- ½ cup cilantro
- ¼ cup tarragon
- ¼ cup dill
- ¼ cup chives
- Juice of 1 small lemon
- ½ cup extra virgin olive oil
- 4 garlic cloves
- 3 green onion bulbs, chopped
- 1–2 ripe avocadoes (or 1 cup frozen and thawed)
- 1 tablespoon capers
- 1 cup arugula or watercress
- 2 cups spinach (optional)
- 1 tablespoon honey (optional)
- ¼ cup water (optional, to thin dressing if too thick)
- ½–1 teaspoon kosher salt, to taste

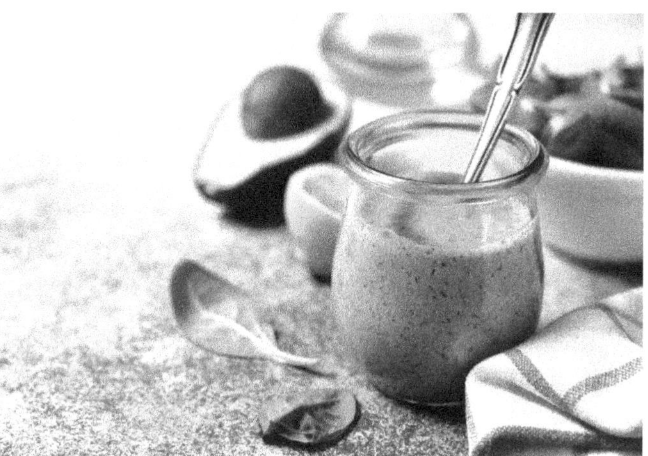

Add all ingredients to a blender, starting with the apple cider vinegar. Placing the liquid in first helps the blender to process the other ingredients easier. Process until smooth. Add water to reach your desired consistency if needed. Season with salt as needed. Store in an airtight container in the refrigerator for up to two weeks.

Makes 4 cups.

LIME CILANTRO DRESSING

- 1 jalapeño pepper, minced
- 1 teaspoon lime zest
- ¼ cup freshly squeezed lime juice
- 2 garlic cloves, minced
- ¼ cup cilantro, chopped
- ½ teaspoon kosher salt
- ¼ teaspoon ground black pepper
- ¼ cup extra virgin olive oil or vegetable oil

In a small bowl, whisk together the jalapeño pepper, lime zest, lime juice, garlic, cilantro, salt, and pepper; then gradually whisk in the oil. Pour over salad or pasta, or use as a marinade for the protein of your choice. Store in an airtight container in the refrigerator for up to one week.

Makes about 1 cup.

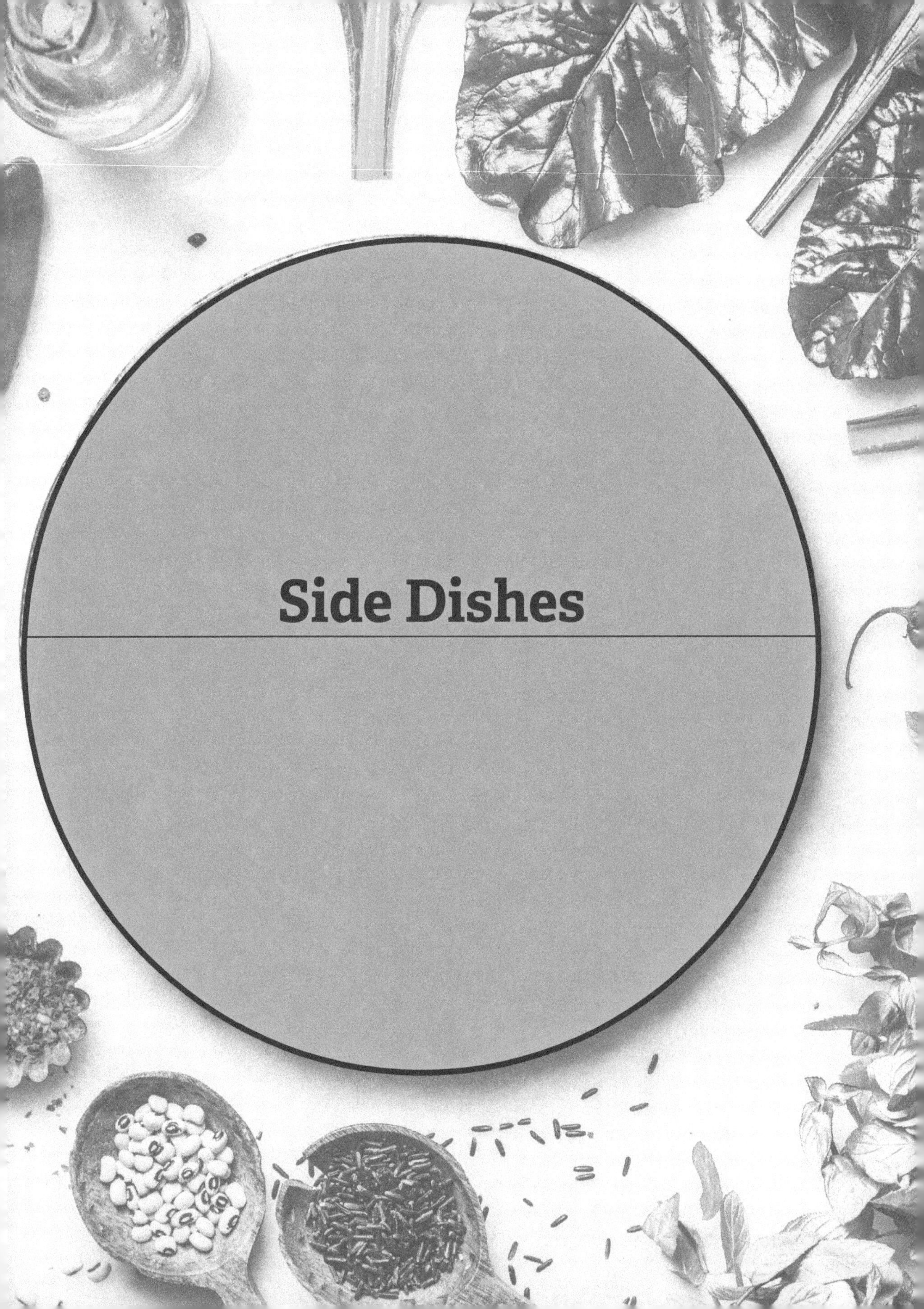

Side Dishes

GRANDMA'S FRIED CORN

When my mom told me this was the recipe for her delicious creamed corn I had been eating all my life, I was a bit confused. Despite its ending as a velvety delight, its beginning involves frying in a skillet for a few minutes. Nonetheless, this recipe was passed down from my grandmother Louise to my mother, who passed it on to me. I hope you enjoy this as much as I do.

- 6 ears of fresh corn on the cob (yellow or white), shucked
- 1 tablespoon flour
- 2 teaspoons salt, divided
- ½ teaspoon ground black pepper
- ½ teaspoon ground mustard (optional)
- ½ stick vegan butter
- 1 tablespoon olive oil
- 2 cups corn broth, added gradually

In a large bowl, cut corn kernels off the cob with a large knife until all kernels are removed. Prepare the corn broth: Break the ears of corn in half. Place the ears of corn in a pot large enough to completely submerge them in water. (You want a yield of at least 2 cups of broth once boiled). If desired, add ½–1 teaspoon of salt to water. Raise the heat until the water is just boiling, cover the pot, and boil for 10 minutes. Remove from heat. Add the flour, salt, black pepper, and mustard to the corn kernels and mix well. Warm a cast-iron skillet over medium heat. Add butter and oil to the skillet. Once the butter is melted and sizzling, add the corn mixture. Stir continuously for 3 minutes. Lower the heat, then add 1 cup of corn broth, stirring constantly. Cover and simmer for 20–30 minutes, stirring every 8–10 minutes. After the corn has been simmering for about 15 minutes, and ½ cup of corn broth and stir. The consistency should be creamy. If not, add the remaining ½ cup of broth gradually until creamy. Serve warm.

Makes 6–8 servings.

VEGAN SOUTHERN BAKED BEANS

The perfect dish for summer days, this recipe is scrumptious as is, but you can add your favorite plant-based ground beef for that meat-like texture. It's sure to be the star at any cookout!

- 3–4 tablespoons extra virgin olive oil
- 1 green bell pepper, diced
- 1 medium onion, yellow or red, diced
- 1 package of plant-based ground beef substitute, optional
- 1 (28-ounce) can vegetarian baked beans, including the bean juice in the can
- ¼ cup ketchup (organic preferred)
- 2 teaspoons yellow mustard
- 1 tablespoon vegan Worcestershire sauce or coconut aminos
- ½ cup dark brown sugar
- Liquid smoke, optional
- Salt and pepper to taste

Preheat the oven to 350°F. Swirl olive oil in a large nonstick skillet a few times. Add the bell pepper and onion and sauté until softened, about 5–7 minutes. Add the ground beef substitute and cook until warmed through, about 3 minutes. Add the beans to a medium baking dish. Add the bell pepper, onions, ground beef substitute, ketchup, mustard, Worcestershire sauce or coconut aminos, sugar, and a few shakes of liquid smoke. Stir until combined. Add salt and pepper to taste. Bake in the oven for 20–25 minutes, or until the edges of the beans start to bubble.

MOMMY'S COLE SLAW

No cookbook of mine would be complete without one of my mother's original recipes! I love this version because it is the perfect combo of sweet, tangy, and crunchy.

- ½ green cabbage, core removed, chopped
- ½ purple cabbage, core removed, chopped
- 1 large carrot, peeled and chopped
- ½ yellow or red medium onion, diced
- 1 tablespoon sugar (then to taste)
- ½ teaspoon of salt (then to taste)
- 2 tablespoons apple cider vinegar (then to taste)
- ¼–½ cup of vegan mayonnaise

Feed the cabbages and the chopped carrot into a food processor using the feed tube, and shred using the shredder blade. Remove from the food processor, place in a large bowl, and add the onion. Whisk together the sugar, salt, apple cider vinegar, and vegan mayonnaise in a separate bowl. Add just enough to the cabbage mixture until everything is coated but not soggy. Serve chilled and store the leftover portion in the refrigerator in an airtight container for 2–3 days.

Makes 6–8 servings.

CHEEZEE VEGAN MAC 'N' CHEEZE

This version of mac 'n' cheese gives the classic comfort food a healthy makeover. If you don't tell anyone this is vegan, they will never know.

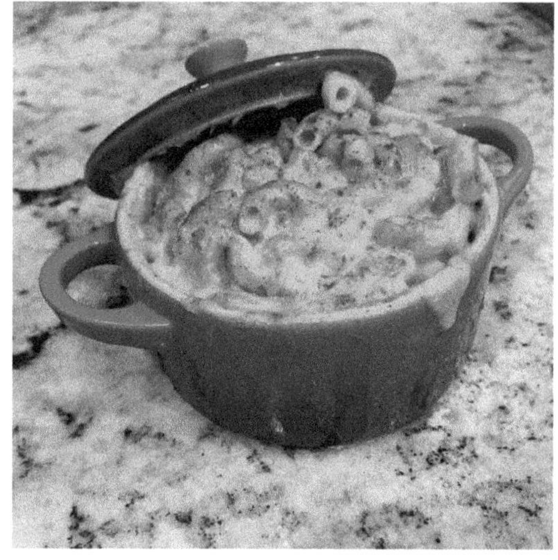

- 2 tablespoons plant butter
- 2 tablespoons whole wheat flour
- 2 cups soy or almond milk
- 3 tablespoons nutritional yeast
- 2 (8-ounce) packages vegan cheddar cheese, divided into 1 ½ cups and ½ cup
- ½ teaspoon smoked paprika
- 1 tablespoon ground mustard
- ½ teaspoon salt
- ½ teaspoon ground black pepper
- 1 tablespoon garlic powder
- ½ box whole wheat elbow macaroni, cooked *al dente* according to package directions, drained well

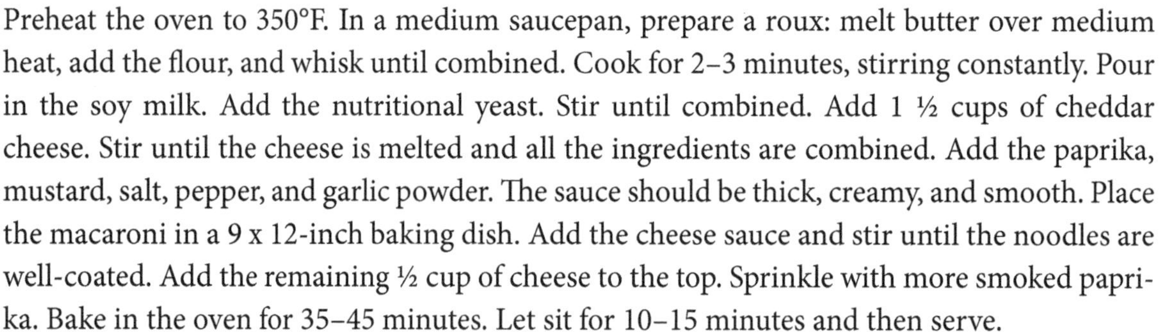

Preheat the oven to 350°F. In a medium saucepan, prepare a roux: melt butter over medium heat, add the flour, and whisk until combined. Cook for 2–3 minutes, stirring constantly. Pour in the soy milk. Add the nutritional yeast. Stir until combined. Add 1 ½ cups of cheddar cheese. Stir until the cheese is melted and all the ingredients are combined. Add the paprika, mustard, salt, pepper, and garlic powder. The sauce should be thick, creamy, and smooth. Place the macaroni in a 9 x 12-inch baking dish. Add the cheese sauce and stir until the noodles are well-coated. Add the remaining ½ cup of cheese to the top. Sprinkle with more smoked paprika. Bake in the oven for 35–45 minutes. Let sit for 10–15 minutes and then serve.

Makes 16 servings.

CILANTRO LIME RICE

- 1 cup uncooked rice (I prefer to use purple, but any rice will do)
- 2 cups of water or vegetable stock
- 1 tablespoon plant butter
- 1 teaspoon kosher salt
- Zest and juice of 2 limes
- Handful of fresh cilantro, chopped

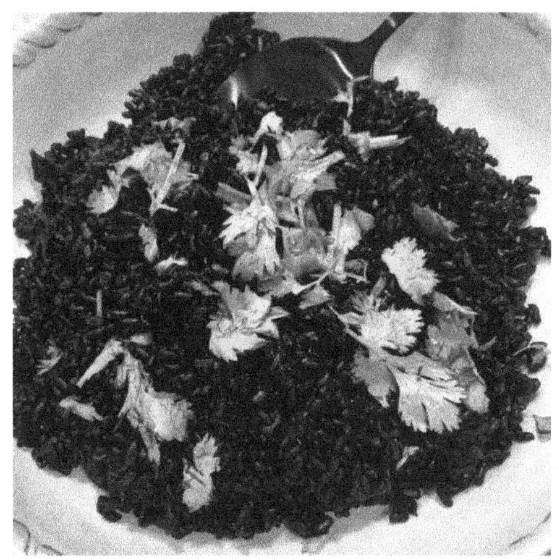

Add the rice, water, butter, and salt to a pot. Cook the rice according to package instructions. Remove from heat when the rice is cooked. Add the lime zest, lime juice, and cilantro to the rice and fluff the rice with a fork. Serve warm as a side dish or in burritos or bowls with your protein of choice.

Makes 8 servings.

NOTES FROM THE LAB

When it comes to side dishes, there are so many directions you can take. Other suggestions include:

- Line a baking sheet with parchment paper, and cover with evenly-chopped vegetables such as carrots, zucchini, eggplant, asparagus, sweet potatoes, or parsnips. Sprinkle with olive oil, salt, and pepper and bake at 400°F until soft, about 35–45 minutes, flipping halfway. Don't be afraid to experiment with spices such as cumin, curry, smoked paprika, etc.
- You can add water or vegetable stock to cooked squash, cauliflower, or potatoes and mash or whip. Use salt and pepper to taste. Miso broth works well, too (just watch the sodium content).
- Serve a simple salad as a side dish, or sticks of fresh vegetables.
- Choose your favorite grain, such as quinoa or millet, or pasta such as couscous, and prepare according to the package directions. Season with salt and pepper and serve with your main course. You can also add vegetables and herbs to give your grain more nutritional value.
- Pickled onions, cabbage, and beets make a nice alternative to standard side dishes.

Use your imagination. You can also serve fruit (including avocadoes, cucumbers, and tomatoes) as a side dish, or vegan apple sauce.

Soups

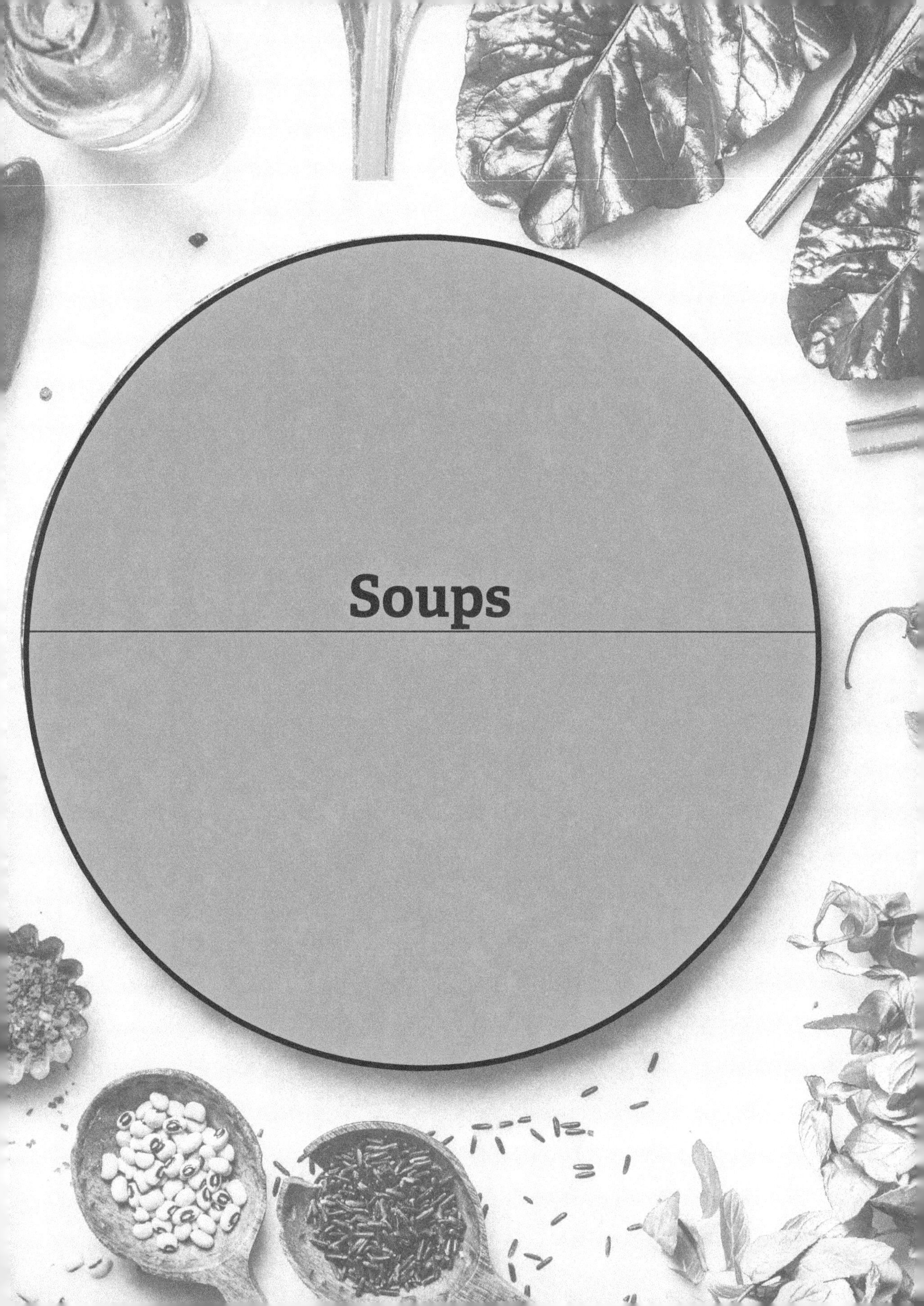

Soups are one of my favorite types of meals for a variety of reasons. They usually require just 1 pot to cook, and they can be a great way to repurpose food, clean out your fridge, or introduce new types of vegetables and plant-based proteins. I love to eat a big bowl of hearty soup (chili included) on a chilly winter night!

VEGAN BLACK BEAN SOUP

- 1 tablespoon olive oil
- 1 large onion, chopped
- 1 celery stalk, chopped
- 2 carrots, chopped
- 4 garlic cloves, chopped
- 2 tablespoons chili powder
- 1 tablespoon ground cumin
- 1 pinch black pepper
- 4 cups vegetable broth
- 4 (15-ounce) cans black beans, rinsed
- 1 (15-ounce) can whole kernel corn, rinsed
- 1 (14.5-ounce) can crushed tomatoes, with juices
- Tortilla chips (optional)

Heat oil in a large pot over medium heat. Sauté the onion, celery, and carrots for 5 minutes. Add the garlic and sauté for 30–60 seconds, until the garlic becomes fragrant. Season with the chili powder, cumin, and black pepper; cook for 1 minute. Add the vegetable broth, 2 cans of beans, and corn. Bring to a boil. Meanwhile, in a food processor or blender, process the remaining 2 cans of beans and tomatoes until smooth. Stir the blend into the boiling soup mixture, reduce the heat to medium, and simmer for 15 minutes. Serve with tortilla chips or over grains like rice or quinoa.

Makes 8–10 servings.

KALE, SAUSAGE, RED POTATO, AND CANNELLINI BEAN SOUP

- 4 teaspoons olive oil divided into 2 sets of 2 tablespoons
- 6 ounces seitan or vegan sausage, chopped
- 1 large onion, diced
- 4 celery ribs, diced
- 8 garlic cloves, minced
- 6 cups low-sodium vegetable broth
- 2 cups water
- 8 ounces fresh kale, thick stems removed, leaves sliced into ribbons
- 12 ounces red potatoes, cut into quarters, with skin left on
- 1 teaspoon smoked paprika
- ¼ teaspoon cayenne pepper
- ½ teaspoon salt
- 1 (16-ounce) can small white beans or cannellini beans, rinsed and drained

Heat 2 teaspoons oil in a large soup pot over medium heat. Add the seitan or sausage and cook until browned all over, about 5 minutes. Remove and place in a bowl. Add 2 more teaspoons of oil and add the onion and celery to the pot; cook until soft, 5–6 minutes. Add the garlic and cook 30–60 seconds, until fragrant. Return the sausage to the pot and add the broth, water, and kale. Bring to a boil over high heat and then reduce heat to medium-low. Cover and simmer until the kale begins to wilt, about 10 minutes. Stir in the potatoes, paprika, cayenne pepper, and salt. Cover again and simmer until the potatoes and kale are tender, 15–20 minutes. Add the beans and cook until they are just heated through, about 5 minutes. Serve with crusty bread.

Makes 8–10 servings.

CARROT SOUP

This is my take on one of the first recipes I made in culinary school. I tweaked it to give it more depth of flavor. Who knew something made from carrots could taste so good?! Perfect for a chilly or rainy day, this soup is pretty satisfying.

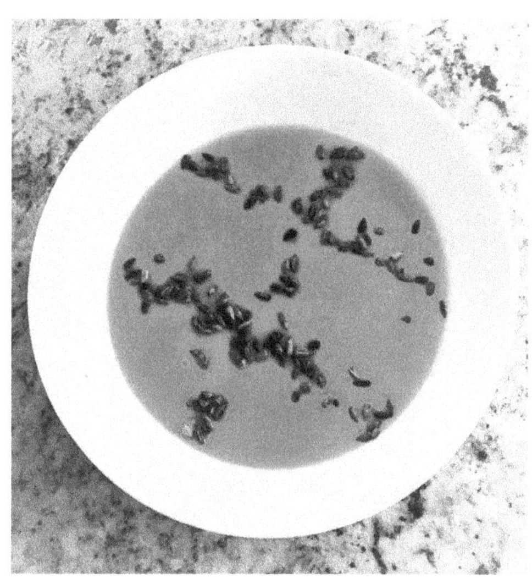

- 2–3 tablespoons olive oil
- 1 pound carrots, small diced
- 1 medium onion, small diced
- 1 teaspoon curry powder
- 1 (1-inch) ginger root, minced
- 2 garlic cloves, minced
- 1 quart vegetable stock or water
- 1 medium sweet potato, small diced
- ½ cup coconut milk, full-fat
- 1 teaspoon kosher salt (then to taste)

In a large saucepot, heat oil over low heat. Add the carrots and onion. Cook until just softened, stirring often, for about 5–7 minutes. Do not let them brown. Add the curry powder and stir just until the veggies are coated. Add the ginger and garlic; cook 30–60 seconds, until aromatic. Add the vegetable stock and sweet potatoes. Bring to a boil and then reduce to a simmer. Cook until the vegetables are soft when pierced by a fork, at least 15 minutes. Remove from the heat and puree the soup in the pot with an immersion blender or in a blender until smooth. Return the soup to a simmer and add the coconut milk. Simmer until warm. The soup should be silky and creamy. Add more stock if needed to reach the right consistency. Serve warm with toasted seeds, croutons, or crusty bread.

Makes 6–8 servings.

GREEK-STYLE CHICKPEA SOUP

This is an example of a hearty Greek dish that is vegan-friendly. Serve with slices of fresh whole grain bread and a salad.

- 3 (15-ounce) cans of chickpeas, drained and rinsed
- 1 large onion, chopped
- 1 teaspoon dried rosemary
- 1 teaspoon sea salt
- 4 garlic cloves, finely chopped
- 1 (28-ounce) can crushed tomatoes (keep the juice)
- 3 cups water
- 2 tablespoons olive oil
- Salt and pepper to taste
- 3 tablespoons fresh, chopped parsley

Add all the ingredients except parsley to a large pot. Bring to a boil, then simmer on low for an hour until the flavors are well blended. You can also cook this soup in a Crock-Pot on the low setting for 4–6 hours. Top with fresh parsley and serve.

CLASSIC MINESTRONE SOUP

This is an all-time favorite of mine. The nice thing about this recipe is that you can use whichever vegetables you have on hand. This recipe can serve as a guide.

- 2 large carrots, peeled and chopped
- 3 celery stalks, chopped
- 1 medium onion, chopped
- 2 garlic cloves, minced
- 2 zucchinis, chopped
- 1 cup broccoli florets
- 1 cup spinach leaves
- 1 can crushed tomatoes
- 1 cup canned kidney beans, rinsed
- 8 cups water
- 1 cup small pasta, such as elbows or orzo
- Salt and pepper to taste
- Fresh chopped parsley for garnish (optional)

Combine all the ingredients except the pasta in a soup pot. Bring to a boil and then simmer for at least 1 hour until the vegetables are soft. Add the pasta during the last 15 minutes of cooking and cook for 8–10 minutes. Garnish with parsley. You can also cook the soup in the Crock-Pot; just add all of the ingredients (except parsley) at once.

MY VEGAN-*ISH* JOURNEY

When I started re-evaluating my food choices and creating healthier recipes, I began to search for ways to "vegan-ize" some common dishes and create new ones. Along the way, I discovered some crucial must-haves, foods, and hacks that have helped me grow my palate and prepare delicious vegan meals. This process allowed me to experiment, create, and test recipes featuring vegetables or other plant-based foods. I also got to create in my lab (also known as my kitchen) while using my many kitchen gadgets and appliances. *Winning!*

Since I also enjoy a good list, I thought I would share my favorite discoveries. These foods have helped me on my journey thus far, and they are presented here in alphabetical order. I call them **Dr. Monique's Favorite Vegan Food ABCs**. This is a behind-the-scenes, "peel-back-the-onion" inside-view of my faves thus far (I just couldn't resist the *corn-y* food pun guys, sorry/not sorry), as well as a look at how some of the recipes in this book came to be.

DR. MONIQUE'S FAVORITE VEGAN FOOD ABCs

A IS FOR AVOCADO

I cannot say enough about this fruit (yes, the avocado is technically a berry because it has fleshy pulp and a seed). I am a bona fide avocadoholic (I even have a T-shirt that says the same)! Avocados are truly a superfood: they contain *lots* of nutrients, fiber, antioxidants such as folic acid, omega-3 fatty acids (the good fat), minerals such as potassium and magnesium, and vitamins such as A, C, D, E, and K. They are also cholesterol- and sodium-free.

Avocados can be used for breakfast (avocado toast, avocado waffles), appetizers, dips (um, guac anyone?), entrées (avocado pasta), and even dessert (chocolate avocado pudding? Yes, please!).

For all their perks, they can be a bit diva-like when it comes to shelf life and storage. Avocados can be high-maintenance but are well worth the effort. To begin, when choosing an avocado, you need to check for ripeness by pressing gently on it. If it is very soft, it is too ripe, so don't waste your money (unless you plan to use it *immediately*—like in the parking lot as soon as you leave the store). Also, the darker the avocado is, the riper it tends to be. Another trick is to check the top of the avocado, where the stem is. If the cap is still on there, flick it off. I use two silly sayings to help remember what to do: "If it's brown, put it down" and "If it's green, it stays on the scene."

I usually buy my avocados unripe (very firm to the touch with no give) and let them ripen on the countertop if I don't plan to use them for a few days. Once they start to ripen, I will store them in the refrigerator to slow down the ripening process. If you want to speed up the ripening process, store your avocado in a paper bag with an apple or banana. The gasses released from these fruits speed up the ripening process (food plus science for the win!). If you eat your avocadoes in halves, be sure to store the unused half with the seed in place, squeeze some lemon or lime juice on it, and cover with plastic wrap to keep it from turning brown. It should last for about a day. You can also freeze avocados whole or squeeze them into ice cube trays. I recommend squeezing fresh lemon or lime juice on them if you do the latter.

Be sure to check out my recipe for **Vegan Avocado Waffles**. Spoiler alert: The avocado takes the place of eggs, giving you a heart-healthy boost as well as beautiful waffles with flecks of green in them from the cilantro. Be sure to bookmark this recipe for St. Patrick's Day. Enjoy!

B FOR BEANS

Black, pinto, red, kidney, garbanzo, lima—the list goes on and on! Did you know that there are over 40,000 types of beans? Beans are part of the legume family, which includes peanuts, alfalfa, clover, peas, chickpeas (aka garbanzo beans), lentils, and soybeans. These little powerhouses are packed with protein, fiber, vitamins such as B, E, and K, and minerals such as iron, calcium, and potassium. They also contain zero fat or cholesterol. Dried beans are also sodium-free.

Canned beans *do* contain sodium, however, so I buy low-sodium or no-salt-added canned beans and rinse them off before cooking them. When it comes down to it, beans check a lot of boxes: these pantry must-haves are economical, versatile, nutritious, easy to cook, and have a long shelf life. They can also be used in a variety of dishes, including appetizers, breakfast, entrées, soups, beverages, and even desserts like brownies! I mean, what would chili be without beans? Vegetarian chili can be just as filling as its meat-containing cousin. And one of my family's favorite recipes is my vegetarian southern baked beans, with just the right touch of sweetness and smokiness and zero meat (but don't tell them that—they still don't know).

I admit that I usually use canned beans, but recently I have started cooking with dried beans. Part of my reluctance to use dried beans before was the time it takes to soak them, which can range anywhere from 1 hour to overnight. (Soaking and rinsing beans are very important in decreasing the chance of developing the gas that can come from eating beans.) Fortunately for me, it was just a matter of time before my love of gadgets and appliances combined in a way that totally changed my mind! I have been "borrowing" my mom's Power Quick Pot (is it still considered borrowing if you never plan on giving it back?), and I discovered that the pressure cooker option has some awesome presets, such as quinoa (my new breakfast obsession!), brown rice, risotto, and yes . . . beans! I tried it for #MeatlessMonday to make a delicious 16-bean medley that I served with plant-based sausage over purple rice. Yum! My seventeen-year-old son even ate *two whole bowls*—and here I was thinking that one bowl would be sufficient. Growing boys and their bottomless-pits-stomachs. Go figure. But I was actually glad that he was eating more plant-based protein instead of animal-based. One disclaimer: I did have to run the cook cycle twice on the Power Quick Pot to get the beans cooked correctly because I had not soaked them first, but it was still faster than if I had cooked them on the stove. This dish makes for a perfect winter's night meal. When using dried beans, remember that a little bit goes a long way: a cup of dried beans yields 2–3 cups of cooked beans, making them ideal for batch cooking as part of your meal prepping.

I do need to give a special mention to black beans, which are probably my personal favorite. I have used them in everything, from brownies to black bean burgers. Black beans are so versatile that my son *still* doesn't know that the brownies he gobbled up one Christmas were actually made from black beans! When they are processed in a food processor, they take on a creamy, fudgy texture that makes a healthy and delicious base for a brownie recipe. I also love them seasoned with cumin, chili powder, and cilantro and served over rice. I could go on and on, but suffice to say, I strongly recommend that you stock your pantry with both dried and canned beans and explore the limitless options they offer as you explore more plant-based meals.

Try my **16-Bean Medley with Plant-Based Sausage and Purple Rice** recipe for yourself!

C FOR CILANTRO

Cilantro is definitely one of my favorite herbs. I discovered it in Mexico many years ago in the *best* pico de gallo I have ever had. I have to qualify this and say the best *restaurant-made* pico de gallo, because of course I think mine is the best I have ever had. Its fresh and citrusy flavor truly transformed my life, and now I use it whenever I can. It is part of the same family as carrots, celery, and parsley. It is also part of the same plant as coriander: the leaves are called cilantro, and the dried seeds are known as coriander. Cilantro is used around the world in African, Caribbean, Chinese, Indian, and Thai dishes. It adds a tantalizing freshness and has a citrus-meets-parsley flavor—to most people. Interestingly, 20 percent of people think that cilantro tastes like soap due to a genetic predisposition.[4] These (unfortunate) people can detect a substance in cilantro that is similar to a compound in soap and stink bugs as well. However, crushing the cilantro before eating the leaves can change this substance into one that is more palatable.

Fortunately, I am not in that group because I cannot imagine life without cilantro! I use it in rice (with lime juice and zest), salsa, guacamole, burritos, quesadillas, vegetable stock, and even waffles! I make a **Mexican Pesto** using cilantro and avocado instead of basil. I just swap out the Parmesan cheese for cotija cheese (grated Mexican cheese, which in its aged form is similar to Parmesan cheese).

Cilantro makes my list not only for its taste but also due to its many health benefits. Because it is so flavorful, extra salt may not be needed. It also contains antioxidants and may be useful in preventing some forms of cancer and infections. Cilantro has essentially no calories and contains potassium, beta-carotene, vitamins C, A, and K, and small amounts of folate (which is important in preventing birth defects).

It may be no coincidence that cilantro goes so well with the first two items on my **Favorite Vegan Foods ABCs** list (avocado and beans). In fact, one day I was inspired to create a dish from some foods in my refrigerator at the time and found that cilantro and beans were the perfect ingredients for my dish. I simply combined some chopped cherry tomatoes, red onion, red and green bell peppers, jalapeño pepper, corn, black beans, lime juice, and cilantro. Served with tortilla chips, this side dish was so delicious I almost ate the whole bowl in one sitting! I call it my **Mexican-Inspired Refrigerator "Clean-Out**." You're welcome!

D FOR DAIRY REPLACEMENTS

Part of the challenge and reward of adopting a more plant-based diet has been finding simple and easy-to-find replacements for milk, cheese, butter, and yogurt (see Chapter 1). My favorites so far, by category, are:

- **Milk:** Soy, coconut, oat, and almond milks. These milk options are unsweetened and are good sources of calcium. They have no cholesterol and very little sodium. Also, they contain no trans fat and either no or very little saturated fat. I use them as 1:1 replacements for any recipe that calls for cow's milk. Coconut and almond milks tend to be a bit creamier than soy, which is more watery.
- **Butter:** Plant butter. I use the Country Crock brand that offers olive oil, avocado, and almond varieties, and I prefer the olive oil one. Speaking of olive oil (although it is not a dairy product), I sometimes use it interchangeably with butter (for sautéing vegetables, for example), but more on olive oil later. I use plant-based butters to make my vegan and gluten-free pound cakes, and I honestly do not miss dairy butter at all! These butters are a blend of plant-based oils, including palm, canola, and olive oil. As such, they do contain small amounts of saturated fats, but no trans fats at all. Saturated fats are considered "unhealthy" and should comprise no more than 10 percent of your daily caloric intake, but eating low amounts is probably okay. Compared to dairy butter, however, plant butter is a much better option. Both saturated and trans fats can raise your bad cholesterol (or LDL as we call it), and as a result, increase your risk for heart disease that can lead to heart attacks. However, trans fats are the most harmful because they also lower your levels of the good, protective cholesterol known as HDL, which decreases heart disease risk. Saturated fats actually *raise* your HDL levels, which is a good thing. Another great thing about plant butters is that they are cholesterol-free. See Chapter 1 for some more information about the pros and cons of using plant butter.
- **Cheese:** Full disclosure here: I was initially not a big fan of vegan cheese due to its bland taste and lack of meltability (if you have tried to melt vegan cheese, you know what I mean). The one brand I do like is Violife. I have tried their cheddar, feta, and

mozzarella cheeses and have been pleasantly surprised. This brand tends to be lower in sodium than some of the other brands. Some brands contain about 10 percent of the recommended daily amount of sodium, approximately 230–240 mg per ¼ cup serving. Surprisingly, the sodium content of some vegan cheeses is actually higher than what is found in the same amount of regular cheddar or mozzarella cheese (but lower than feta). Since I have high blood pressure, I am always on the lookout for hidden "salt bombs" (foods that are unexpectedly high in sodium). In addition, some vegan cheeses can be highly processed with chemicals that can be hard to pronounce. They are cholesterol-free, though, which is good. Violife tends to melt easier as well. Another substitute for cheese is nutritional yeast. It is vegan, gluten-free, and loaded with B vitamins, including B12 (if fortified), thiamine, niacin, riboflavin, and folate. It has no cholesterol and almost no sodium (only 10 mg per tablespoon). Nutritional yeast can add umami (read: savory or meaty) flavor. Umami is one of the five taste profiles (the others are sweet, salty, bitter, and sour), so to have a vegan replacement option is more than ideal. Nutritional yeast can be added to a variety of foods, such as macaroni and cheese, sauces, popcorn, pizza, and baked potatoes, to name a few. I am so excited to add this ingredient to my repertoire and further explore what I can do with it! More on nutritional yeast later.

- **Yogurt:** Greek yogurt gets an honorable mention here because it has more protein and less sugar than regular yogurt. Traditional Greek yogurt is made with goat's milk, whereas the American version is made with cow's milk, placing it squarely in the vegetarian category. I use it in my **Handful Smoothie**. I call it that because I literally add a handful of spinach, a handful of frozen fruits (berries, pineapple, mango, etc.), and a handful of frozen riced cauliflower (which adds fiber and makes you feel full without affecting the taste), along with other ingredients including flaxseed and plant-based protein powder. It is a creamy, refreshing, nutrient-filled smoothie, perfect after a workout or as a meal replacement. However, I recently found a recipe for a vegan alternative and made some yogurt myself. Raw cashews, lemon juice, and apple cider vinegar in a blender and voila! It was so easy that I was inspired to make my own recipe. If you are just starting on your vegan journey or are looking for new dairy alternatives, give some of these a try!

E FOR EGG SUBSTITUTES

As discussed in Chapter 1, eggs serve various purposes in so many dishes that replacing them can be quite challenging for those embarking on a vegan journey. They are used in everything from breakfast to dessert. In baking (which I do a lot of), they add structure, height, flavor, and moisture. In addition to that, in savory dishes (like quiche), they also serve as a thickener and help hold everything together. So, the challenge (and the rewarding payoff once you figure out what works best) is finding the right egg substitute for the intended dish. So far, these are the ones I have discovered and have either used or plan to use very soon. Please note that this list is not all-inclusive, just the ones that I prefer.

- **Applesauce**: Applesauce is low in calories and contains helpful antioxidants. Unsweetened, organic applesauce adds moisture to cake and quick bread batters. Use ¼ cup applesauce for each egg you are replacing. I also use cinnamon-flavored applesauce in my sweet potato cakes or pumpkin vegan pound cakes. Applesauce can also be used to replace oil in baking as well.
- **Flaxseed**: Ground flaxseed is a very good source of omega-3 fatty acids, which decrease the risk for heart disease and stroke. It is also rich in lignans, which are antioxidant substances that decrease the risk of cancer such as breast and prostate. Lastly, flaxseed also contains a lot of fiber, which is important for colon health, can lower cholesterol, and improve blood sugar control. Flaxseed is used to create the fleggs that feature prominently in this book. Substitute 1 egg with 1 heaping tablespoon of ground flaxseed mixed in 3 tablespoons of water. Let the mixture sit for at least 10 minutes in the refrigerator until it becomes viscous or egg yolk-like. I whisk mine to introduce air, which can help make baked goods a bit fluffier. On a side note: flaxseed is also good to add to smoothies, oatmeal, quinoa, granola, and salad dressings.
- **Silken tofu:** Tofu is made from soybeans. It contains proteins, minerals such as iron and calcium, and like other items on this list, antioxidants that help boost your immune system. Tofu also helps to lower LDL cholesterol, prevent breast and prostate cancer, and reduce hot flashes in postmenopausal women. Silken tofu works well as a binding agent in desserts. The substitution is ¼ cup per egg.
- **Apple cider vinegar (ACV) and baking soda**: ACV has antibacterial properties and can also help lower blood sugar in diabetics. The substitution math here is easy: for each egg, use 1 tablespoon of vinegar (apple cider is my fave) and 1 teaspoon of baking soda. The resulting chemical reaction helps to make cakes and quick breads rise. In my recipe for **Mitchell's Vegan and Gluten-Free Chocolate Cake**, I use ACV and baking soda, as well as flaxseed, for a fluffy, moist, delicious cake.
- **Yogurt:** Plain yogurt can be used in muffins, cakes, or cupcakes. Use ¼ cup per egg. Keep in mind that yogurt adds moisture, so you may need to bake for an extra few

minutes; it may be a better option for brownies. Keep in mind, this is a vegetarian option, not vegan, unless of course you use vegan yogurt.

- **Aquafaba:** The next time you open a can of chickpeas, don't rinse the liquid down the drain. Aquafaba is the liquid in a can of chickpeas (or any can of beans) and is used as a substitute for egg whites. It can be used unwhipped or whipped (like in a meringue). Use 3 tablespoons per egg called for in a recipe. Aquafaba acts as a binder in baked goods and is also used in homemade mayo or aioli.
- **Carbonated water:** Surprisingly, carbonated water adds moisture to baked goods and also makes them light and fluffy due to the air bubbles. Ideal for use in cakes, cupcakes, and quick breads, use ¼ cup to replace each egg.

Mitchell's Vegan and Gluten-Free Chocolate Cake recipe was inspired by my son Mitchell and sells out when I take it to the farmer's market. This cake is chocolatey, moist, and 100 percent delicious!

F FOR FRESH AND FROZEN FRUITS AND VEGETABLES

Okay. This is a no-brainer—it's not exactly breaking news that fresh fruits and vegetables are good for you. There is not much to be said that you don't already know about the benefits of eating fresh fruits and vegetables. They have no labels to read and decipher. They are environmentally friendly due to their lack of packaging. Lastly, they are considered whole foods because they are not processed. All that aside, they are also just visually appealing. I cannot tell you how much pleasure and excitement I get when I walk into the produce section of my grocery store! The varieties, colors, and combinations are limitless. Fresh fruits and veggies are chock-full of antioxidants, anti-inflammatories, vitamins, minerals, protein, fiber, good fats, and complex carbs. Factor in that some varieties are either at their peak seasonality or available only at certain times of the year (like butternut squash or strawberries), and that trip to the store can make you feel like you have stumbled upon a gold mine.

But let's face it—most of us do not have the time, resources, or desire to go to the grocery store 3–4 times a week in search of fresh produce. Unfortunately, due to social distancing, slower production, and shipping issues caused by COVID-19, finding your faves at the market may be challenging, or even worse, more expensive than before. In fact, it's times like these when I really wish I had a green thumb and could grow my own produce. . . . *sigh* . . . maybe one day. But here is where frozen produce comes in handy and saves the day. Frozen options make it possible to enjoy your favorites year-round and may even give you access to varieties that may not be available to you locally.

Frozen fruits and vegetables are usually picked at their prime. They are picked when they are ripe. Fresh vegetables can then be blanched (placed in boiling water briefly and then placed in an ice bath to stop the cooking process, which preserves the color and texture as well as certain nutrients) before being frozen, often in a location close to the field from which they were harvested. Because of this process, frozen vegetables may actually contain more vitamins and phytonutrients (beneficial chemicals produced by plants) than the fresh produce at the grocery store. Another reason why frozen may be better than fresh has to do with how much time has elapsed since the food was picked. The produce in your supermarket may have traveled quite a ways to get to you, or it may have been sitting in the store for a while and may not be at its peak freshness anymore. This time delay can decrease the actual amount of vitamins and beneficial plant chemicals the produce contains by the time you buy it. Interestingly, the amounts of carbs, protein, minerals, and fiber they contain are not affected, so fresh and frozen produce have the same amounts of these nutrients.

If you are fortunate enough to get your produce from your local farmer's market, travel time would not be an issue. The farmers or their representatives can tell you when their produce was picked. Some chain grocery stores offer local farmer's market produce, which should be pretty fresh. Ask the grocery manager what day their deliveries from local farms arrive so you can time your shopping trip.

A newer option for obtaining fresh produce is to sign up for a subscription box, which will deliver fresh produce to your door. There are a variety of options, including organic and "ugly" vegetables that may not sell in grocery stores due to aesthetic imperfections. Purchasing a subscription box may be cheaper than shopping from your local grocery store, and some services use recyclable cardboard boxes.

A word about organics: Organic produce, by definition, is free from pesticides, genetically modified organisms (GMOs), and harmful hormones. In my opinion, sometimes it also tastes better than non-organic produce. However, organic produce is usually more expensive (and smaller) than conventionally grown produce. If you want to buy more organics but are looking to save on your grocery bill, you can pick and choose the items for which you shell out the extra bucks. Generally speaking, if you will be eating the skin or outermost layer of the fruit, opt for organic. Strawberries, peaches, green beans, sweet bell peppers, carrots, and sweet potatoes are a few examples. Apples, lettuce, and broccoli are considered to be low risk for having high levels of pesticides, so those that are grown conventionally should be okay to buy. However, you may want to opt for organic for some produce grown in the US. Be sure to wash all produce thoroughly before eating. You can make a simple produce wash by adding 1 part white vinegar to 3 parts water. Place the produce in a clean sink and soak for about 5 minutes. Rinse well, dry, and prepare as desired. This works well for fruit (like apples) that you want to have easily accessible for healthy snacks. For most veggies, wait until you are ready to use them because washing them and then storing them can make them spoil faster. For leafy greens, wrap them in clean paper towels or cloth towels, and then store them in a zippered plastic bag or an airtight container.

As for frozen fruits, I enjoy having my choice of frozen mango, pineapple, berries, and avocado (remember, avocado is a fruit). Making smoothies with frozen fruits is super easy, and they add color, nutrition, ice, and bulk. Frozen fruits do not undergo the blanching process described above for vegetables, so they do not lose any of the water-soluble (meaning they dissolve in water) vitamins they contain, such as B vitamins and vitamin C. Be sure to look for sales and consider buying frozen fruits at warehouse stores to save on the price. If you do buy in bulk, before you freeze them at home, break them down into portions that make them easier to use. Using sandwich bags or ice cube trays helps with portion size. Be sure to label and date them and keep the FIFO approach: first in, first out. This means that you use the items that have been stored the longest before using fresher ones.

If you plan on freezing your own produce (whether you grew it in your garden or bought some in bulk), be aware that not all produce is freezer-friendly. A general rule of thumb to keep in mind is that if it has a high water content, it will not do well when defrosted or thawed. Fruits like watermelon, strawberries, and oranges are best kept and used while frozen, like in a smoothie or blended drink. Vegetables that are best to avoid freezing and then thawing include celery, cucumbers, lettuce, and radishes. They will become limp and soggy if you do so. Instead, use them frozen in dishes like soup or casseroles, which can be more forgiving than, say, a sauté or stir-fry (I think it's best to use fresh, crisp vegetables for the latter).

Bottom line: However or wherever you get your produce, whether it be fresh from your garden, delivered in the mail, at your local farmer's market, or in your grocery store produce aisle or the freezer section, be sure to get anywhere from 5 to 13 servings of fruits and vegetables per day. Try to get as many different colors as you can to get all the antioxidants, vitamins, and minerals that you deserve and that your body craves! My recipe for an easy **Fresh Fruit Salad** topped with fresh mint will help you reach your daily goal!

G FOR GINGER AND GARLIC

I gotta tell ya, these two are definitely in my personal top five when it comes to seasoning my food. Garlic (which is actually a vegetable) and ginger (a spice) add flavor and depth to my kitchen creations and make my kitchen smell like a 5-star restaurant. Fresh ginger and garlic can be found in any grocery store, and fortunately, they are both pretty inexpensive. Their ground versions are also widely available and affordable as well. In addition, they have many health benefits that belie the small amounts that are typically used in a recipe.

Garlic: Millions of people around the world, on pretty much every continent (not too sure about Antarctica), from many different cultures and countries, *cannot* be wrong. Garlic is used in so many different types of cuisines for many good reasons. Some of my favorite Caribbean, Italian, Chinese, and Indian dishes feature garlic as a key ingredient. Don't take my word for it: Pause for a moment and think of your favorite or most memorable dish from a foreign vacation. Chances are pretty good that garlic played a role in creating the happy times your taste buds experienced and that you may have been trying to recreate ever since.

Garlic is in the same family as onions, shallots, and leeks (to me, a shallot tastes like the love child of onion and garlic). In addition to its high-flavor profile, garlic makes my favorites list for its many health benefits, some of which are listed below:

- Contains many minerals and vitamins, and has antibacterial, antiviral, and antifungal properties
- Has anti-inflammatory properties
- May lower both your total cholesterol and bad (LDL) cholesterol levels, which may decrease the risk for heart attack
- May reduce risk of lung cancer
- May reduce hip arthritis
- May decrease the frequency of the common cold

To use fresh garlic, invest in a sharp chef's knife if you have great knife skills, or if you are knife-challenged (like me), then a garlic press, Microplane grater, or box grater are other options. Quick cooking tip: When sautéing minced garlic in combination with other vegetables (for example, green bell pepper and onion), be sure to add it in after the vegetables have cooked sufficiently (usually about 5–7 minutes), and then cook for only about 30–60 seconds, which is the amount of time it takes for the garlic to become fragrant. Cooking garlic for too long will make it burn and ruin your dish. Don't forget to use a good-quality extra virgin olive oil so that the fresh taste of garlic shines through. Roasting garlic gives it a slightly sweeter taste due to the caramelization of the natural sugars. Mash up the roasted, softened garlic and add it to butter to make your own garlic butter. One of my favorite garlic-featuring recipes, **Fresh Basil Pesto**, is versatile and easy to make. This restaurant-quality condiment can be used on sandwiches, pasta, or protein of any kind.

Be sure to store fresh garlic in a cool, dark place, preferably in a clay pot with holes. Whole garlic bulbs can last for months, but individual cloves may last for only about two weeks.

Okay, I know what you're thinking: prepping fresh garlic can be messy, what with the papery outer leaves that fly around everywhere and the smell of garlic on your hands after handling it. All that drama may make you want to buy minced garlic from the store. Believe me, I've been there. But the drawback is that jarred garlic is made with citric acid to prolong shelf life. If you have a (mini) food processor or a sharp chef's knife, you can easily make your own minced garlic to have on hand for recipes. All you need is some extra virgin olive oil, a bunch of garlic, and a small glass jar (I recycle glass jars of all sizes). All you have to do is chop up the garlic, place it in a glass jar, add enough oil to cover it, and seal tightly with the lid. Stored properly, it can last for several weeks in the refrigerator.

Ginger: Like garlic, ginger is used in many different cuisines and has many health benefits as well. However, unlike garlic, ginger can be used in both savory dishes and desserts. It can be grated, chopped, juiced, and even candied. It should be stored in the refrigerator, unpeeled, in a resealable plastic bag. I also freeze my ginger for longer storage. I buy it in bulk, rinse it off, pat it dry, and place it in a resealable storage bag. When I need it, I just use my Microplane to grate what I need and add it directly into my recipe (the same trick works for turmeric root as well).

Some of ginger's health benefits include:

- Can be used to fight nausea (think ginger tea or ginger ale) and motion sickness
- Anti-inflammatory effects on joints
- Antioxidant effects, which means it protects your body's DNA and decreases the risk for chronic diseases like high blood pressure and heart disease
- Antimicrobial and antiviral properties
- Immune system boosting
- Appetite booster
- Helps relieve upper respiratory infection symptoms

I love the combo of garlic and ginger, and when I make Asian-inspired dishes (like my **Cauliflower Rice Stir-Fry with Duck Sauce and Hot Mustard** or vegan pot stickers), this dynamic duo, plus plenty of scallions (aka green onions), gives those dishes an authentic taste.

H FOR HERBS

First, let's clear up a common area of confusion: What *is* the difference between herbs and spices? Both add flavor and depth to dishes, and both come from plants. But herbs are the actual leaves of the plant, while spices come from the roots, bark, and seeds. Fresh herbs are so fragrant and elevate any meal, so I use them whenever I can. Fresh cilantro, basil, mint, dill, rosemary, tarragon, and thyme are my absolute favorites. Chives, lemongrass, and sage get honorable mentions as well. That being said, my spice rack is full of dried herbs that I certainly use in heavy rotation.

Given that they are green plants, it should be no surprise that herbs have many health benefits.

Let's review just a few:

- **Basil**: has antioxidant and anti-inflammatory properties, which decrease the risk for chronic diseases such as cancer, heart disease, and arthritis; lowers blood pressure, cholesterol and blood glucose; antibacterial; can improve anxiety and depression and decrease the risk for memory loss related to aging.
- **Cilantro**: has antioxidant properties; is full of fiber, and has minerals such as potassium, iron, and calcium, B vitamins (including folic acid), and vitamins A, C, and K.
- **Dill:** has antioxidant, anti-inflammatory, and antibacterial properties; contains vitamins, and minerals important for healthy bones such as calcium, magnesium, and phosphorus.
- **Mint:** has antioxidant and anti-inflammatory properties; freshens breath; relieves abdominal pain and irritable bowel syndrome.
- **Tarragon:** has antibacterial properties; contains potassium.
- **Sage:** contains antioxidant vitamins A, C, E, and K; contains minerals (magnesium, copper, zinc); may help lower blood sugar.
- **Lemongrass:** helps relieve upset stomach, headache, upper respiratory infection symptoms; improves skin and hair; has antibacterial and antioxidant effects.
- **Chives:** may help prevent cancer, osteoporosis, and memory loss.

A quick word about storing your fresh herbs: dirt and moisture can make them wilt quickly. For herbs sold in bunches, when you bring them home, untie them and rinse them in cold water. Wrap them in damp paper towels and refrigerate them in a resealable bag. For basil, trim the stems and place them in 1 inch of water and store them on your countertop, away from direct sunlight. If you grow your own herbs or buy them in large bunches, most of them can be frozen to prevent them from going bad. Dust off those ice trays and place the herbs in each cube section and then drizzle in olive oil. Place in an airtight bag and freeze for 6–9 months.

Keep in mind that dried herbs are more potent than fresh, so a tablespoon of fresh herbs equals a teaspoon of dried. Add dried herbs at the beginning of your cooking and add fresh herbs at the end or after cooking, especially the more fragile herbs, such as basil and cilantro. Sturdier herbs, such as rosemary and thyme, can be added much earlier in the cooking process.

My recipe for **Dr. Monique's Mango Muddled Mint Mock Mo-garita**, a refreshing, colorful drink, features fresh mint. Get transported to a tropical island while drinking a glass full of nutrition—and of course, if you want to make it an "adult" beverage, enjoy responsibly!

I FOR INDIAN SPICES

The letter *I* was a bit more challenging—all I could think of was ice cream, and a Google search yielded a lot of exotic foods I had never even heard of (like imarti and icaco). And then it hit me! The best part of my vegan-*ish* journey has been trying new ingredients or using familiar ingredients in new ways. This of course includes fresh herbs and ground spices. My spice cabinets (yes, plural, because one is just not enough) have long-held bottles of cumin, curry, coriander, cinnamon, nutmeg, paprika, turmeric, cloves, fennel seeds, ginger, and cayenne pepper, but I have recently begun experimenting with them in Indian food-inspired combinations. So, *I* is for Indian spices!

True story: It is *soooo* funny how the universe works. Once I came up with the topic for the letter I, I still needed some background and most definitely a mouth-watering recipe to share. Well, a few nights before I wrote this, I had some wonderful butter chicken with garlic naan (two of my absolute favorite Indian foods). Earlier that day, I had seen a video on social media featuring someone using king oyster mushrooms in place of pork for BBQ ribs. Whoomp! There it was! Clearly, I was meant to create a vegan butter chicken recipe using these glorious mushrooms! I had tried making a vegan butter chicken recipe using tofu several weeks prior. While the flavors were definitely there, I admit the textures were not quite what I wanted, so the idea of trying it again using a hearty mushroom was very intriguing!

In addition to the spices I have already mentioned, I have also fallen in love with other Indian staples such as cardamom and fenugreek. Green cardamom (not to be confused with black cardamom, which has a completely different taste) has a lovely sweet and lemony taste, and I use it in my vegan lemon pound cake recipe. It is also part of the seasoning trio that is known as garam masala. Literally meaning "warm spice mix," garam masala is a mixture of ground cinnamon, cardamom, and cloves. Of course, I have made my own mix using my spice grinder (kitchen gadget junkie here, remember?). I store it in a recycled glass spice jar, labeled and dated so that I remember what it is and when I made it. In fact, as I sit here writing this, I am sipping on some green tea that I added garam masala to in a tea infuser. It reminds me very much of the mulling spice that I add to apple cider, except with a twist of citrus that goes well with honey. It makes me feel warm and cozy inside, the perfect drink on a chilly day.

As for any health benefits these spices may have, not only are they good tasting, but they are also good for you. A few honorable mentions:

- Cardamom: has antioxidant and anti-inflammatory properties and may help fight bad breath and prevent cavities.
- Fenugreek: may help increase the amount of breast milk produced by lactating women and encourage weight gain in infants. Can improve testosterone levels and sex drive in men. May help lower blood sugar and cholesterol.
- Coriander: comes from the same plant as cilantro (the seeds are called coriander and the leaves are called cilantro). Contains antioxidants and has antibacterial properties. It may reduce blood sugar, bad cholesterol, and high blood pressure, but more human studies are needed.
- Cinnamon: has antioxidant and anti-inflammatory properties. Also has antibacterial, antiviral, and antifungal properties. Helps with digestive issues and may reduce blood pressure and blood sugars (however, more formal studies are needed to answer this question definitively).
- Nutmeg: also has antioxidant and anti-inflammatory properties, as well as antibacterial effects. May help boost libido and improve mood but human studies are needed to know for sure.
- Cloves: have antioxidant and antibacterial properties. May also help lower blood sugar, but again, more studies are needed.
- Fennel seeds: have antibacterial and antifungal qualities, help to reduce inflammation, and help relieve constipation.

With all of these health benefits and the wonderful aromas they provide, Indian spices are a wonderful, healthy way to add flavor to meat substitutes such as tofu, tempeh, seitan, and mushrooms. When cooking with these and other spices, I find that I do not have to use much salt, which is good for anyone with hypertension (high blood pressure) such as myself. I use just enough salt to help the flavors come together in perfect harmony.

My **Vegan "Butter Chicken"** recipe features king oyster mushrooms as the chicken substitute. It is a bit of a misnomer because there is no butter or chicken in this recipe (am I the only one reminded of the hilarious Linda Richmond character on *Saturday Night Live*? I can still see her patting her ginormous hair while saying: "Rhode Island is neither a road, nor an island. Discuss, discuss!"). However, the oysters provide the perfect chicken-like texture, and the sauce is luxurious while being lighter and guilt-free when compared to the original recipe that is made with butter.

J FOR JACKFRUIT

Jackfruit is the largest tree fruit in the world, and one fruit can weigh up to one hundred pounds! They are indigenous to South India and are related to figs and mulberries. Due to their size and sticky quality, fresh jackfruit can be a bit intimidating to cut up and prepare, so I prefer to use the ready-to-eat canned version instead. Fresh jackfruit has a subtle sweet and fruity flavor, similar to apples, bananas, pineapples, and mango. It has been said that it tastes similar to Juicy Fruit gum.

In all honesty, the first time I tasted canned jackfruit, I did not like it. It was in a BBQ recipe that was quite bland, and I wasn't crazy about the texture. But I had to take my own advice. I am always encouraging my followers to try new things (#TryItTuesday or #WonderWednesday) or to try old favorites in different ways. So, I decided to give jackfruit another try, just made my way. And guess what? I loved it! I have used it in "crab" cakes, curry, and of course, "pulled pork" recipes. It can also be used as a substitute for pulled chicken. Another plus is that canned jackfruit is relatively inexpensive, costing about $2 per can. Some stores stock it in plastic bags in the frozen section; that type is better used in fruit smoothies or desserts due to its sweeter taste.

Canned jackfruit has a somewhat plain taste, which means that you can season it however you like: with curry, BBQ, or Creole seasoning, to name a few. They all work because jackfruit is a blank canvas on which you can create whatever you choose. You can even play with the texture and size of it. When I use it in my faux crab cakes, I place it in my food processor and pulse just a few times. It then looks just like lump crab meat. When I use jackfruit as a stand-in for pulled pork, I like to sauté it first for 10–15 minutes to dry it out and toughen it up a bit. By drying it out this way, it makes the flesh more "meaty" and pork-like in texture.

Nutrition-wise, jackfruit really packs a punch. It is rich in antioxidants such as vitamin A and vitamin C. Vitamin A is important for eye health, and vitamin C helps protect the skin from harmful effects from the sun. It also has a lot of B vitamins. Jackfruit contains minerals such as potassium and magnesium, which are important for bone, muscle, and nerve health. In fact, adequate potassium intake can lower blood pressure and decrease the risk for stroke and heart attack. Jackfruit also provides a good amount of protein despite being a fruit, approximately 3 grams per cup.

Like any other fruit, jackfruit has plenty of phytonutrients, which are beneficial chemicals made by plants. These phytonutrients may help prevent diseases such as cancer, macular degeneration of the eye, and heart disease. Jackfruit may also help diabetics control their blood sugars. Since jackfruit is actually absorbed and processed by the body slower than other fruits, diabetics will not see their blood sugars go up as high. This is due to its low glycemic index (GI), which is a number on a scale of how high your blood sugar will rise after you eat something containing carbohydrates. Foods with a low GI do not cause your blood sugar levels to rise too high too quickly after being eaten, typically within two hours. Diabetics who eat a lot of jackfruit should watch their blood sugars carefully. If they are on any medications, it is possible that their doctor may need to decrease the doses to prevent their levels from dropping too low from the combination.

My recipe for **Pulled "Pork" with Homemade BBQ Sauce** is super easy to make from ingredients you likely already have at home. Of course, it is much healthier than what you buy in the store (read: *high fructose corn syrup*) and can be tweaked however you like. Want it spicier? Add ground cayenne pepper or fresh jalapeño or habanero peppers. Smokier? Add more smoked paprika and liquid smoke. Tangier? Add more vinegar.

K FOR KALE

Truth be told, people tend to be in one of two camps when it comes to kale. They either hate it, or they love it. I, fortunately, am in the latter camp. Kale is a member of the dark leafy green vegetable family. As such, it is ridiculously good for you and has tons of health benefits. It is also a wonderful ingredient in smoothies, soups, casseroles, salads, and of course, kale chips. It can be used wherever you use collard greens or even spinach. Kale comes in many different varieties. Soft-textured varieties, like baby kale, can be eaten raw. Varieties with tougher leaves, like common curly kale, need to be cooked or marinated after removing their tough stems in the middle.

Kale is actually in the same cruciferous family as broccoli, cabbage, brussels sprouts, and cauliflower. It is loaded with essential minerals and vitamins, including iron, copper, magnesium, and calcium. Calcium is important for healthy, strong bones. As a leafy vegetable, it should be no surprise that kale is full of fiber. Fiber makes you feel full, which decreases the urge to snack. Fiber also helps to keep your bowels healthy and in good working order. Kale contains antioxidant vitamins, such as vitamins A and C. In fact, kale has more vitamin C than its other leafy green vegetable cousins. One cup of kale actually has more vitamin C than an orange. Kale also contains a large amount of vitamin K, which is important for people who take blood thinners such as warfarin (brand name Coumadin) to know. Large amounts of kale and other leafy vegetables can affect the blood-thinning effect of this medication, so people taking warfarin have to be careful and be sure to get their blood levels monitored regularly.

As a member of the cruciferous vegetable family, kale has plant-based compounds that help to decrease the risk of certain cancers. In addition, its fiber helps to decrease the risk of colon cancer. Kale also helps to lower cholesterol levels in the body, which decreases the risk for heart disease. The high levels of beta-carotene, which your body converts to vitamin A, help protect your eyes and decrease the risk of macular degeneration and cataracts. Vitamin C is important for a healthy immune system and helps your joints as well.

As mentioned above, kale leaves can be made into chips! I just rinse them, pat them dry, toss them with a little bit of olive oil, season them with kosher salt and freshly ground black pepper, and bake them in the oven at 250°F for about 20–30 minutes. I do check on them around 15 minutes to make sure they're not getting done too quickly or burning.

My **Kale, Sausage, Red Potato, and Cannellini Bean Soup** is a hearty soup that is full of flavor and nutrition, and the fiber it contains goes a long way in filling you up and keeping you warm on a cold winter's day. Be sure not to omit the smoked paprika; it really brings out the flavor!

L FOR LENTILS

Lentils are one of my newer discoveries on my vegan-*ish* journey. I have had them in various dishes at restaurants (CAVA, I'm talking to you!), but I have just recently begun cooking with them. Out of the many varieties to choose from, my favorites are brown lentils and black lentils. Keep in mind, there are many others to experiment with, including red, yellow, and green. The type of dish you are making determines which lentil you should choose. For example, some lentils hold their shape better and can be used in salads (like black lentils) or as meat replacements (brown or green lentils). Others (like red lentils) get soft when cooked, so they are better when added to curries, soups, or stews.

Lentils are part of the legume family and are powerhouses of nutritional value. They contain zero fat and cholesterol and are very low in carbs. They are packed with B vitamins, magnesium, and potassium. They are also protein-rich, making them a very good meat substitute. In addition, they contain quite a bit of iron.

The fiber content in lentils helps promote bowel health by aiding with healthy bowel movements. In addition, because they are a member of the plant family, they have phytonutrients and anti-inflammatory effects that help to decrease the risk of chronic diseases such as heart disease and type 2 diabetes. Lentils also help to decrease the risk of certain cancers such as colon, prostate, and stomach cancers. Lentils may help with weight loss due to the feeling of fullness after eating them, which cuts down on snacking between meals.

In my honest and humble opinion, lentils really should be in every pantry: they are extremely inexpensive and can be found alongside dry beans in your grocery store. They have a long shelf life and are very easy to cook, requiring no soaking like dry beans. You just need a pot, water (or a seasoned stock), and seasoning of your choice. However, you do want to be sure to inspect them for any stones or debris that may be in the package. Simply place them in a pot, add water (the rough rule of thumb is 2–3 cups of water for each cup of lentils), seasoning, and a tiny amount of salt. Bring them to a boil, then allow them to simmer. Cover them and cook for 15–20 minutes to the desired consistency of your choice. In order to stop the cooking process, drain and rinse them in cold water.

A word of caution: eating large amounts of lentils can increase the risk for flatulence and bloating. If you are new to the lentil game, I suggest you gradually increase your intake over time, so it won't overwhelm your digestive system. People with irritable bowel syndrome (IBS) may want to speak to their doctor first or if they have any symptoms after eating lentils. In people with IBS, lentils may actually cause constipation.

I use lentils as a binder in my **Red Rice, Brown Lentil, and Mushroom Burger**. I created this recipe after spending $15 for a vegan burger at an Atlanta hotel. I took one bite and the whole darn thing fell apart! Needless to say, I was disappointed, so I decided to make one myself. If necessity is the mother of invention, then frustration must surely be its father! I whipped this burger recipe up in the lab and placed it on the grill for those beautiful grill marks. I placed it on a bun and topped it with fixings just like I do for a traditional burger (adding avocado slices to replace the mayo). If you want to skip carbs, you can wrap it in lettuce instead of buns. It is delicious and filling, and it doesn't fall apart!

M FOR MAPLE SYRUP

After several savory discoveries, it's exciting to talk about something sweet! My approach to desserts is *everything in moderation*. I don't want to live in a world where I can't have dessert from time to time. And that is not what adopting a healthy lifestyle is about in my opinion. I personally do not believe in eliminating all enjoyable food items from one's diet. I just encourage people to find healthier ways to enjoy their favorite treats and "dessert responsibly." My go-to sweetener for several of my baked goods is maple syrup. Let me just start by saying: all maple syrup is *not* created equally. The maple syrup that I use and will be referring to is 100-percent maple syrup, not to be confused with imitation maple syrup or maple-flavored syrup. The latter is made with high fructose corn syrup, artificial flavors, and chemicals. The difference between the two is significant. The maple syrup that I'm referring to is produced from actual tree sap. It is one of my preferred sweeteners in baking or even in my **Tablespoon BBQ sauce** recipe. Maple syrup comes in different grades. Here in the US, we have either grade A or grade B syrups, and they can vary by color: light, medium, or dark. Interestingly, the tree sap that is harvested later in the season is used to produce a darker-colored syrup and has a more robust maple flavor (grade B, for example).

Now, do not be misled: maple syrup *does* contain sugar, and as such, should be used in moderation. It does also contain beneficial nutrients such as antioxidants (the darker syrups have higher levels) and minerals like zinc, calcium, and iron. In addition, maple syrup has a lower GI than regular table sugar. Remember, the GI is a number indicating how quickly a food containing carbohydrates will elevate your blood sugar levels after you eat it. The lower the number, the better. The GI for maple syrup is 54, compared to 65 for table sugar. Unfortunately, maple syrup essentially does not contain vitamins.

Bottom line: If you are going to use maple syrup *instead* of sugar, just be aware that you are still eating sugar and should do so in moderation. Maple syrup may have a very slight edge over table sugar but should not be considered "healthy" (like, say, a vegetable would be). It just may be less harmful overall for you. Diabetics should definitely monitor their blood sugars closely when eating maple syrup.

That being said, I choose to use maple syrup in my baking recipes because I can use less of it than refined sugar. The ratio is ⅔ cup of maple syrup for each cup of sugar. I use it as the sweetener in my **Vegan and Gluten-Free Sweet Potato Pound Cake with Maple Orange Glaze**. It goes without saying that cake should be eaten in moderation so that you are not eating excessive calories on a regular basis. For example, I usually make this for special occasions, like Thanksgiving.

The way I describe my **Vegan and Gluten-Free Sweet Potato Pound Cake with Maple Orange Glaze** is if a sweet potato pie and a pound cake had a baby, this would be it! Flavored with cinnamon, nutmeg, and vanilla, it goes well with a cup of tea or coffee.

N FOR NUTS

Let me start by saying I truly feel sorry for those who are allergic to nuts! They add so much extra flavor to everything they are added to that I cannot imagine life without them. That being said, for those of us who can enjoy them, let's deep-dive into the health benefits of a variety of nuts. We will also briefly mention seeds as well. Adding just a handful of a variety of nuts to your diet will boost your health in several ways. There are many different varieties of nuts, but for this discussion, I will focus on Brazil nuts, almonds, cashews, walnuts, and pecans.

Quick side note: Peanuts are not actually true nuts. They are members of the legume family, which makes them cousins to peas and lentils, so they will not be included in this discussion. Just a word about peanut allergies: The nuts that will be discussed here—Brazil, pecan, walnut, etc.—are considered tree nuts, and people who have peanut allergies can also be allergic to these nuts as well, so they should proceed with caution.

So where do I start singing the praises of nuts? There are many health benefits to eating nuts. For example, they are packed with antioxidants, contain no cholesterol, and are high in minerals. Nuts are a good source of protein, and they contain many substances that are good for your heart, such as unsaturated fats (the good kind of fat), fiber, and omega-3 fatty acids. One downside is that they are high in calories, but when eaten in moderation, they have not been shown to increase weight gain. Remember, when we talk about how many daily servings of nuts you should get, that includes a few tablespoons of various nut butters, such as almond butter or cashew butter.

Let's take a crack at each one individually (sorry, I had to do it) and look at their health benefits:

Almonds:

- Contain prebiotics (fiber that gut bacteria feed off of), which help to restore the healthy bacteria in your gut.
- Increase your good cholesterol (HDL) and lower your bad cholesterol (LDL).
- Can help prevent skin aging.
- Contain a large amount of fiber, as well as vitamin E and vitamin B.
- Contain minerals such as calcium, iron, and potassium.
- Can be made into almond milk and almond butter.

Brazil nuts:

- Contain many vitamins, including B vitamins and vitamin E. Vitamin E is an antioxidant that decreases your risk for heart disease and cancer.

- Contain the minerals calcium, iron, potassium, and zinc, all essential for the normal functioning of your brain, heart, muscles, and immune and nervous systems.
- Contain a lot of healthy fats as well.
- Are a good source of the mineral selenium, which is important in keeping your thyroid healthy and helping your immune system to work.
- Fun fact: The cool thing about Brazil nuts is that you only need two per day to get the recommended selenium intake. Not two cups, handfuls, or even tablespoons. Just two little nuts. More than four or five can actually cause selenium poisoning.
- Help improve bone density due to their magnesium levels.

Cashews:

- They are rich in fiber and protein, which are needed for healthy bowel function and muscle building, respectively.
- They contain minerals such as copper and iron. These minerals play key roles in heart function, nervous system function, healthy, strong bones and muscles, and blood cell production.
- They may be lower in calories and may help with weight loss.
- Cashews are also a staple in vegan cooking as they can be soaked and processed into creams and sauces. They can even be used to make vegan yogurt and vegan sour cream.

Pecans (my personal faves):

- They contain protein, healthy fats, and fiber. They are also a good source of iron, potassium, and magnesium.
- Contain a good amount of copper, which is an important mineral in immune system function, bone marrow production, red blood cell function, and nervous system function.
- Contain zinc, which supports your immune system and helps wounds to heal.
- Pair very nicely with maple syrup for a tasty, sweet snack.

Walnuts:

- Are rich in antioxidants (more so than other nuts), such as vitamin E, which helps with gut health.
- Help decrease inflammation and may help with brain function and decrease the risk for Alzheimer's disease. Coincidentally, the grooves and crevices in walnuts look similar to the surface of the brain, so it makes sense that they are brain food!
- May help reduce certain types of cancer such as breast prostate and colon cancers.
- May help lower blood pressure and thereby decrease the risk for stroke and heart attack.

Honorable mention: Seeds like chia, flax, sesame, pumpkin, and sunflower have a lot of the same health benefits as nuts and are a better option for people with nut allergies. I sometimes use sunflower seeds as a substitute in my pesto instead of pine nuts. They decrease bad cholesterol, blood sugar, blood pressure, and appetite. They can be used to make healthy snacks and can be added to smoothies and salads just like nuts can. In fact, when mixed with water, both chia and flax seeds serve as egg replacements. Hemp seeds contain all of the essential amino acids (meaning the ones your body cannot make) and are a very good source of protein.

Nuts and seeds can be used in a variety of recipes. For example, if you want to bump up the flavor and fiber content of your morning bowl of oatmeal (or, in my case, quinoa), toast up some pecans or walnuts and toss them in. Don't forget to add them to salads for extra crunch, along with dried cranberries and crisp Gala apple slices. Toasting nuts on the stove brings out their flavor even more and makes them a welcome addition to baked goods or cereals.

My **Vegan Blondies** recipe features pecans. These are made with—surprise!—*navy beans* for a totally vegan experience. The liquid in the navy bean can, aquafaba, is used as the egg replacement in this recipe. The pecans add a nice bit of texture and compliment the butterscotch flavor as well. Just like black beans can be used to make moist, delicious brownies, this vegan version of a blondie magically turns beans into an addictive treat. In case you are wondering, blondies are made with vanilla and brown sugar instead of the chocolate used to make brownies.

O FOR ORANGES

Honestly, I feel like I'm not even trying with this one. I mean, what's not to like about oranges? They are sweet, juicy, and seem to always be in season. Citrus fruits even have their own handy packaging (just be sure to rinse them off before peeling them). For this discussion, oranges are holding it down for the entire citrus family, which includes lemon, limes, grapefruits, and pomelos, which are the largest member of the citrus family. Lemons and limes add depths of flavor and brighten a variety of dishes, such as marinades, seafood, desserts, etc. Seriously, what is a cup of hot tea or a glass of water without a lemon wedge for added taste?

Citrus fruits, in addition to being downright juicy and delicious, range in taste from sweet to tart. They have tons of health benefits and multiple reasons to be featured prominently in one's diet. As are many of the items on my ABC favorites list, citrus fruits are rich in fiber. They are also very high in vitamin C, which by now you have learned is an antioxidant. Vitamin C helps decrease the signs of aging and helps support your immune system. Vitamin C also helps in the absorption of iron, so people who are anemic are encouraged to increase their citrus intake for this reason and wash down their iron pills with a glass of OJ.

The high fiber content helps your digestive tract work optimally and prevents constipation. You can also eat these fruits guilt-free because they are low in calories. They also contain other beneficial plant chemicals, phytochemicals, that have anti-inflammatory and antioxidant effects. They may help prevent cancer and protect your heart as well. They also may decrease your risk of kidney stones.

True story about fruit juice: When my son was young, my mother was concerned that he wouldn't drink fruit juice. Interestingly, my son only ever drank formula, and then as he got older, milk and water. Somehow, my son must have known intuitively that drinking juices that are high in sugar is actually not good for kids. (*Smart kid. His mom must be a doctor.*) But seriously, like so many people, my mother thought that as a child he needed to drink juice in order to be healthy. Despite my reassurances to her that he was fine without drinking juice, she still was very concerned about this. However, drinking fruit juice increases the risk for cavities as well as weight gain in children. Even 100 percent fruit juices are not ideal because you don't get the amount of fiber you would from eating the fruit itself.

Although citrus fruits are ubiquitous, they are not meant for everyone. Those who should avoid citrus are people who suffer from gastroesophageal reflux disease (GERD, or acid reflux) because citrus can aggravate those symptoms. The other warning about citrus fruit you need to know about is that grapefruit can interact with certain medications, specifically cholesterol-lowering medications, as well as some blood pressure and allergy medications. If you are a grapefruit juice drinker, be sure to discuss with your doctor what medications you should be cautious about.

Lastly, don't throw those citrus rinds away just yet! Grab a Microplane or a box grater (using the small grater side) and get busy making a tablespoon or three of fresh citrus zest. Zest is easily obtained from the rind of citrus fruits. By using these gadgets to take off just the colored part of the rind, you can add so much flavor to your food. You want to be careful not to grate it too deeply (to the white part) because that can be bitter and not taste good. Zest also has health benefits since it contains antioxidants and is good for your immune system, a healthy heart, and may even have antimicrobial and antifungal properties. It is easier if you zest your fruit before you cut it.

My **Homemade Orange Juice** is made with kiwi, cantaloupe, ginger, Gala apples, and navel oranges. I simply combined them in my newest kitchen appliance, my juicer, and made this delicious, freshly squeezed juice from scratch. The fresh ginger adds a nice bit of zing!

P FOR PORTOBELLO MUSHROOMS

Mushrooms are edible fungi, and portobello is just one of many. While your initial reaction may be, "*What? Yuck! I'm not eating that!*" I promise you, portobello mushrooms are some of the ones that are actually good for you. Portobello mushrooms can be quite large. Their meaty caps (or the tops of the mushroom) make for a wonderful meat replacement, as they can be grilled, sautéed, baked, used in sandwiches, etc. They are the larger version of the baby bella mushroom (also known as cremini mushrooms).

How do I love portobello mushrooms? Let me count the ways! Clearly, if they have made this list, that means they are good for you. They are low in sodium, have no cholesterol, and they contain B vitamins such as thiamine, riboflavin, niacin, vitamin B6, and folate. Your body needs a regular supply of B vitamins from your diet because it is unable to store most of them, such as niacin and vitamin B6. Vitamin B12 is the exception since it can be stored in the body for up to five years. Mushrooms also contain the minerals phosphorus, potassium, copper, and selenium.

Let's see why these are important:

- Selenium is important for the health of both your immune and nervous systems. It is also used to make thyroid hormones and antioxidants.
- Mushrooms are a good source of copper, which is also important for healthy immune and nervous systems. Copper helps your body make the connective tissue that holds it together. It is also needed to make blood cells and certain hormones.
- B vitamins help the body in a variety of ways, such as blood cell production, hair and nail growth, and healthy brain function. Niacin helps your body to metabolize (or break down) food. Vitamin B6 helps strengthen the immune system and is needed for the production of brain chemicals called neurotransmitters, such as dopamine and serotonin. These play a major role in mood stabilization.

- Mushrooms are also a very good source of protein and antioxidants, which decrease the risk for chronic diseases such as heart disease, Alzheimer's, and cancer.
- Portobello mushrooms contain small amounts of vitamin D, which is important for immune support, healthy lungs, and strong bones by helping you absorb calcium.
- Portobello mushrooms are a good source of plant fiber and are low in carbs. This is a bonus because you can add them to meals to help you feel fuller without excess carb intake.
- Portobellos are also a good source of amino acids, which are the building blocks of proteins.

Due to their firm texture, portobello mushrooms hold up well when sautéed, baked, or grilled. This feature makes them one of my favorite go-tos when I want a meatless meal. Special shout out to king oyster mushrooms for the same reason, which I use in my **Vegan "Butter Chicken"** recipe.

To clean your mushrooms, rinse them very briefly under running water. You can also wipe them with a damp towel or cloth to get off any residual dirt. Mushrooms have quite a bit of water content that comes out during cooking, and they tend to absorb a lot of water, so you don't want to add excess water by soaking them. Pat away any excess water so they won't become too soggy when you cook them. It is also recommended that you remove the gills when cooking portobellos. The gills are those dark membranes that are on the undersurface of the cap. They are not harmful to eat, but their dark color can make your dish not as pretty as you would like. Just scoop them out with a spoon to remove them.

Portobello mushrooms can be used in salads, stir-fries, and casseroles such as lasagna. Another bonus for portobello mushrooms is that they cook pretty quickly on the stovetop. They really just take a few minutes to sauté, which makes them great for adding them to a quick omelet in the morning. They can also be used as a pizza topping or a filler for tacos, quesadillas, or fajitas. I even use them in my vegan burgers.

A word of caution for people with gout or kidney stones: be sure to discuss adding mushrooms to your diet with your doctor. They should be eaten in moderation since they contain something called purines. Purines are a chemical that the body uses to make the genetic materials DNA and RNA, as well as uric acid. Uric acid is a chemical that, when eaten in excess, will cause gout, which is painful joint swelling, usually occurring in the big toe. Excess uric acid levels can also be harmful to people with kidney disease.

My **Philly Cheeze "Steak" Sandwich** recipe features portobello mushrooms. I attended Temple University School of Medicine in Philadelphia, and during my four years there, I *defi-*

nitely ate more than my share of cheesesteaks. This recipe is my version of one of those iconic sandwiches. Simply sauté the mushrooms with some onions and bell pepper, season them with herbs de Provence (which is a mixture of rosemary, thyme, oregano, and marjoram), and then top with (vegan) provolone or mozzarella cheese. This sandwich can hold its own with the meat version, *periodt!* Unlike the meat version, however, you don't have to worry about cholesterol (depending on whether you use vegan cheese or not) because portobello mushrooms do not contain any cholesterol.

Q FOR QUINOA

I am super excited to write this section because quinoa is *hands down* one of my new absolute faves! Backstory: I have texture issues, and by that, I mean I don't like the way certain foods feel in my mouth. I know, sounds weird, right? For example, I simply cannot stand the way oatmeal feels in my mouth, which is unfortunate because oatmeal is extremely good for you. But the texture just does not work for me. I knew I had to find a healthy alternative for a hot cereal instead of the Cream of Wheat I grew up eating, which can be high in simple carbohydrates and low in fiber content. Enter quinoa to save the day! I have been so happy to discover quinoa that I must spread the word. It is my go-to for a nice, hot, filling breakfast (and of course, it can be used in savory dishes as well).

Quinoa (pronounced keen-wah) has many health benefits and is a good source of protein, carbs, fiber, iron, calcium, and minerals such as iron, potassium, calcium, phosphorus, and magnesium. It contains vitamin E and B vitamins. In fact, it is one of the few plant sources of complete protein (the other is amaranth, another ancient grain gaining in popularity). This means it contains adequate amounts of all nine of the essential amino acids that our bodies cannot make on their own. Essential amino acids should be eaten every day, so they must be a part of your daily diet. Keep in mind that there are twenty amino acids in total that your body needs to function (they are considered the "building blocks" of proteins), but there are only nine that are considered essential. In addition to making proteins, amino acids are used to make hormones and neurotransmitters, which are brain chemicals that affect mood.

Quinoa is actually a seed but is classified as a whole grain. Known as a pseudocereal, it is a seed that is prepared and eaten like the cereal grains wheat, rice, and oats. Quinoa comes in different colors, such as red, white, and black, and you can buy them in mixed bags with all three sold together. My favorite go-to, however, is the white variety (because it is more versatile in my opinion), but red is a close second. I know what you are thinking. My usual advice is to eat your colors, but there are exceptions to every rule, right? Being a member of the plant family, quinoa contains antioxidants and anti-inflammatory properties, which are important in preventing cancer and other chronic diseases such as heart disease and diabetes.

Quinoa contains 30 grams of carbohydrates per ¼ cup, so be mindful of that. However, these are predominately complex carbs that are better for you because they are digested more gradually. This means that they do not cause spikes in your blood sugars like simple carbohydrates do. These spikes and subsequent crashes can cause hunger and irritability and may lead to excess snacking and weight gain.

Quinoa is high in fiber, which plays an important role in bowel health. Fiber helps you feel full, which can lead to decreased snacking and result in weight loss. Quinoa is a good option for people who are gluten intolerant because it is gluten-free. Because it is also high in protein, it can boost your metabolism, which means you burn calories efficiently throughout the day.

I have used quinoa in dishes for breakfast, lunch, and dinner. I add cinnamon, nutmeg, maple syrup, and a splash of vanilla for a warm and hearty breakfast. I also created a **Chocolate Quinoa** recipe for my son, who absolutely loves it—it's like eating dessert for breakfast! I also use quinoa in my **Quinoa and Mushroom Stuffed Peppers**.

R FOR RICE

Rice is a no-brainer. No food list would be complete without rice. It is eaten in many cultures around the world, including African, Asian, and Latin American, for many good reasons. It is easy to prepare, very affordable, and has a long shelf life, making it the ideal pantry staple. According to Ricepedia, "rice is the staple food of more than half of the world's population—more than 3.5 billion people depend on rice for more than 20 percent of their daily calories."[5]

There are two main types of rice: white rice and brown rice (or whole grain rice). Brown rice is definitely the healthier option of the two, as it is not processed like white rice is. Due to processing, white rice is lower in fiber and nutritional benefits than brown rice.

Both white and brown rice are mostly carbohydrates, so if you are watching your carb intake, you may want to try the new plant-based rice substitutes that are available. Cauliflower rice is easy to make at home with a food processor, or you can buy it frozen. Use it just like you would rice, like in my **Cauliflower Rice Stir-Fry with Duck Sauce and Hot Mustard** recipe. Brown rice has many subtypes, including purple, red, and black. Brown rice still has the bran (or outer seed coat), which is high in fiber. It is an unprocessed whole grain and has many more health benefits than white rice. My personal faves are brown, purple, and red rice. I also enjoy basmati and jasmine varieties, particularly in Indian-inspired dishes. There are also rice substitutes made from lentils or chickpeas.

Health benefits of brown rice (and its subtypes):

- Brown rice has a lower GI than white rice, which means it raises blood sugars less than white rice. This is important for diabetics and for decreasing the risk of diabetes that can be seen with white rice in general.
- As a whole grain, it has all the benefits you would expect. Whole grains lower cholesterol and decrease the risk for stroke, heart disease, and type 2 diabetes.
- Purple rice is high in antioxidants, which decrease the risk for heart disease and certain cancers.
- Purple rice also contains several B vitamins that are important for healthy muscles and nerve and heart functions.
- Brown rice contains the minerals selenium and magnesium. Selenium is important in hormone function, especially for the thyroid, and magnesium helps with blood pressure control.

It goes without saying that rice is quite versatile and can be served as a main dish or added to soups, casseroles, stir-fries, etc. It can be cooked using various methods, including using a pressure cooker, rice cooker, or just on the stovetop. Both pressure cookers and rice cookers use steam, but pressure cookers also use pressure as the name implies, and they cook rice much faster. This is key when cooking whole grain rice, which takes longer to cook than white rice. Rinsing the rice first removes excess starch, which results in fluffier rice. One-pot meals are another great dish option because the rice cooks along with everything else and makes cleanup a breeze. One busy weeknight, I made beans and rice in my pressure cooker using my **16 Bean Medley with Plant-Based Sausage and Purple Rice** recipe. For my meat alternative, I chopped up some seitan I had in my freezer and seasoned it all with onion powder, garlic powder, and bay leaves. Thirty minutes later, I had a delicious and filling one-pot meal that is one of our favorites!

A word of caution about rice and arsenic: Both brown and white rice may contain this trace element, which over time can increase the risk for chronic diseases such as cancer and diabetes. To decrease the risk, rinse the rice first and cook it in plenty of water (like pasta, instead of the 2:1 water-to-rice ratio we typically use).

My **Cilantro Lime Rice** works as a side dish but can also be used in a burrito or as the base for a veggie bowl with your choice of protein, roasted vegetables, and other hearty toppings.

S FOR SWEET POTATOES

I absolutely love sweet potatoes! I use them in everything from sweet potato pancakes to candied sweet potatoes, as well as my sweet potato pies and my **Vegan and Gluten-Free Sweet Potato Pound Cake** that we have already discussed.

Sweet potatoes are generally healthier for you than white potatoes, not to mention tastier. One cup of sweet potatoes contains 27 grams of carbohydrates versus 37 grams for white potatoes. This is important because that means that the GI of sweet potatoes is usually lower than the GI of white potatoes. However, baked sweet potatoes have a higher GI than boiled ones because of what happens during the baking process. The glycemic index is the measure of how much a food raises your blood sugar. Diabetics need to be especially aware of these numbers when trying to control their blood sugars.

Sweet potatoes come in many different colors, including white, orange, and purple. Those that are orange are high in beta-carotene, an antioxidant that our bodies convert to vitamin A. Vitamin A helps improve your eyesight, strengthens your immune system to help you fight infections, and is good for healthy skin. Vitamin A is also important for preventing eye diseases such as macular disease, degeneration, and cataracts. Purple sweet potatoes also have beneficial phytonutrients called anthocyanins that help prevent diseases such as cancer and high blood pressure. They may also boost memory.

Sweet potatoes are high in vitamin C, which is also an antioxidant, as well as potassium and fiber. Like other foods we have discussed previously, sweet potatoes help you feel full and can keep cravings and snacking at bay due to their fiber content. This may result in a lower number on your bathroom scale when you weigh yourself. The anti-inflammatory benefits of sweet potatoes are due to their high vitamin content. Because of their anti-inflammatory and antioxidant properties, they may also help decrease the risk of developing chronic diseases such as diabetes. Sweet potatoes also promote gut health from their fiber content and by increasing the growth of "good" gut bacteria.

I created my **Sweet Potato Hash** using some leftover sweet potato french fries that were in my freezer. I added diced bell peppers and red onion and threw them all in my cast-iron skillet, along with some thyme, rosemary, and smoked paprika. This is one of my favorite breakfast recipes; it is a little bit sweet, a little bit smoky, and very filling.

T FOR TOMATOES

Tomatoes are another pantry staple that I recommend everyone should have on hand. They are the ideal pantry-mate because they are inexpensive, have a long shelf life, tend to be low in sodium, and can be used in a variety of dishes. I keep tomatoes of many forms in my cabinet.

I have tomato paste, tomato sauce, and diced or whole tomatoes. Having different options really helps to keep the creative juices flowing (bad food pun intended).

Pop quiz: Are tomatoes fruits or vegetables? If you chose fruit, pop your collar because you are correct! Tomatoes are actually fruits because they come from a flower and contain seeds. That means other "vegetables" that we eat are actually fruits, such as avocado, peppers, and squash. I know—mind blowing, right?

Tomatoes offer many health benefits. In general, tomatoes are high in water content, which makes them so juicy. They contain lycopene, which is a phytonutrient and antioxidant that may help decrease the risk of cancers, particularly prostate, lung, and stomach cancer. They are also a great source of fiber. They contain the antioxidant vitamin C, which is important in immune and skin health. Tomatoes also contain the antioxidant beta-carotene, which gives them their orange color and is converted into vitamin A in your body. This is helpful for healthy eyes and immune function. Vitamin A also helps keep your bones healthy as well. Tomatoes also contain a good amount of potassium, which is important for cardiovascular health and blood pressure control. So, show your heart some love, and add a tomato or two to your meals today!

Tomatoes come in a variety of colors, including red, yellow, orange, and green, and different colored tomatoes offer different health benefits. Yellow tomatoes contain a group of antioxidants that help reduce the signs of aging. Orange tomatoes are high in vitamin E, which can help with inflammatory skin conditions such as psoriasis and eczema. Red tomatoes can actually protect your skin from sun damage due to their high lycopene levels. And green tomatoes (often served fried in the South) are a good source of vitamins A and C, as well as potassium. Like their red counterparts, they also contain essential minerals such as iron, calcium, and magnesium. Although rare, tomato allergy is indeed a thing, and people who are allergic to grass pollen and latex have a higher chance of being allergic to tomatoes. Tomatoes can also aggravate acid reflux or GERD, so people who have this condition may want to eliminate or minimize their tomato intake. This includes tomato sauces as well.

Of the fresh varieties, I enjoy tomatoes in all their forms: cherry, grape, plum, beefsteak, you name it! Fresh plum tomatoes are great for making pico de gallo. San Marzano tomatoes are a variety of plum tomatoes that I keep cans of on hand as well. They are great for making your own pasta or marinara sauces. Sun-dried tomatoes are another option for your tomato repertoire. These are wonderful for adding depth to salads or sandwiches. However, be sure to read the labels carefully to watch for excess sodium. Sun-dried tomatoes may also be higher in calories and sugar than regular canned tomatoes or fresh tomatoes due to the drying process. But it is good to have some on hand to toss on homemade pizza, salads, or sandwiches. Surprisingly, canned tomatoes are one of the few processed foods that I recommend. Canned tomatoes actually contain higher amounts of lycopene than their fresh counterparts due to how they are processed. This is true for ketchup as well. However, be mindful that many ketchup products are made with high fructose corn syrup. You want to avoid that and opt for organic versions instead.

In fact, my thick, delicious **Tablespoon BBQ sauce** was created after I realized that the BBQ sauce in my refrigerator contained high fructose corn syrup, an artificial sweetener linked to obesity, diabetes, and heart disease. Using a whole 6-ounce can of tomato paste, I just added tablespoons of just about every other ingredient until I came up with this concoction. I use a version of it on my **Pulled "Pork" with Homemade BBQ Sauce** and anywhere else I need BBQ sauce. The beautiful thing is it can be tweaked to suit your taste, whether you prefer yours smokier, sweeter, or spicier.

U FOR UNSALTED FOODS

Let's shine the spotlight on salt, or more specifically, *unsalted* foods. Salt (or sodium chloride, its chemical name) has been around since 6,000 BC. Its properties as a preservative have made it very valuable as well as ubiquitous. And yes, it certainly brings out the flavor in food—surely I'm not the only one who likes to add a little salt to apples, watermelon, and cantaloupe to bring out the sweetness? But salt is used very liberally in prepared and processed foods nowadays, even in things you may not suspect. For example, did you know that poultry producers add salt to raw chicken to boost the flavor and make it weigh more? Salt attracts water, which adds to the weight, so that means you pay on average $1.50 extra per package just for added saltwater.[6] Both the health and financial implications of this are more reasons to consider a plant-based diet. Salt can be hidden in a lot of processed foods like pizza, sausage, sandwich meats, fast food, and canned goods.

As someone with hypertension, I personally do not cook with a lot of salt, and I am very careful to read food labels to see how much added sodium is in my food. The recipes in this cookbook are made with very little, if any, added salt. I encourage my readers to look for other healthy and natural sources to flavor your food. Fresh herbs and spices are delicious ways to boost flavor without adding extra salt. Salt is hidden in food labels under a variety of names, such as "natural flavors," sodium bicarbonate, baking soda, baking powder, MSG, sodium, disodium, trisodium, sodium citrate, and sodium nitrite, just to name a few.

So other than making food taste good and satisfying your salty snack cravings, what does sodium do in your body? Sodium chloride is important in the body for normal nerve, muscle, and heart function. The cells of your nervous system use salt to communicate with each other and transmit signals. Salt plays a role in controlling blood pressure as well. For a healthy balance, the recommended amount of salt intake is less than 2000 mg per day (about a teaspoon of table salt), but the ideal amount is 1500 mg. However, in the US, we often exceed that amount (about 3,500 mg per day), particularly by eating a lot of takeout, restaurant, or processed foods, which can easily have more than a day's worth of sodium in one meal.[7] This is bad for you because excessive amounts of salt can cause fluid retention and swelling, increase your blood pressure, and increase the risk for heart attack and stroke. For those with heart failure or kidney or liver problems—or any condition that causes you to have fluid balance issues—you should speak to your doctor about what your recommended amount of salt should be per day.

All salt is not created equally and there are many different types. During my research, I came across an interesting article that said that almost 80 percent of people that were surveyed had at least three different types of salt on hand, and 20 percent had five or more varieties.[8] I actually have several on hand myself: iodized, kosher, sea salt, and black lava. As I mentioned, I am very careful about adding extra salt when I cook. But salt can be hidden in foods and may be sabotaging your efforts to watch your salt intake. My personal experience with this happened about fifteen years ago. I was at a church function and ate some taco soup. It didn't taste salty to me, so I didn't give it a second thought. Well, later that night, I noticed that my hands and feet were very swollen and tight. As I thought about what could have caused this, I realized that the taco soup was probably prepared with some packaged seasoning and ground beef that were both loaded with salt. I realized then that I had become salt-sensitive, meaning that the extra salt had made me retain fluid and caused the swelling in my hands and feet. The extra fluid can make the heart and kidneys work harder. This is why one of the first things we tell people when they are diagnosed with high blood pressure (or to prevent them from even developing it) is to cut back on sodium intake in order to decrease the risk for heart attack and kidney failure.

As you experiment with other ways to season your food, you may realize that you may not even need as much salt as you used to, and after cutting back on salty foods for just one or two weeks, you can actually reset your taste buds. Afterward, foods will likely taste saltier to you than they did before. Keep in mind that one teaspoon of kosher salt, often used for savory cooking, and one teaspoon of table or iodized salt do not equal the same amount of actual sodium. In terms of sodium content, a teaspoon of table salt equals one and a quarter teaspoon of kosher salt, because table salt is smaller and finer than kosher salt, which is coarser and larger. Also, condiments such as ketchup and soy sauce can contain large amounts of sodium. Coconut aminos is a much lower sodium-containing ingredient that can be used in place of soy sauce.

Another way to lower your salt intake is to look for low- or sodium-free options. While the salt content may not be zero, it should be a lot less than what the regular version of that item contains. When you are using any food that is not made fresh, it's going to contain some sodium to help preserve it. Rinse canned vegetables off to remove as much sodium as you can. But of course, the best way to avoid excess sodium is to cook with more fresh fruits and vegetables and season with herbs and spices.

So how can you tell if you are retaining fluid from excessive salt intake? As I mentioned above with my experience, you may notice that your rings are difficult to remove because your fingers are swollen. When you get undressed, if you notice that your socks are leaving an indentation around your calves, that can be a sign of fluid retention (also known as edema). If you notice that you are gaining weight rapidly and don't think it's coming from what you are eating, or if you are having problems sleeping flat at night due to shortness of breath, see a doctor immediately because these are symptoms of fluid overload and could be due to weak heart muscle.

In summary, salt plays a vital role in our bodies, but too much can cause harm and increase the risk for heart attack and stroke. Look for other ways to season your food so you can cut back or even eliminate the need for the saltshaker on your table.

V FOR VEGAN MEAT REPLACEMENT OPTIONS

This topic has definitely been interesting to write about because it has led to quite a bit of experimenting on my part. Typically, when I thought of meat replacements, the first things that came to mind were tofu and mushrooms. However, recently I have discovered other options such as seitan ("wheat meat") and tempeh, which are plant-based meat substitutes. They each have their pros and cons, and it is always good to have a variety of options to choose from when one is trying to swap out meat for a healthier alternative.

Let me share what I have learned about each one (because sharing is caring, right?).

Tofu

Tofu is made from soy and comes in a variety of textures, from silken tofu, which is commonly used as an egg or dairy replacement or in desserts, all the way to extra-firm tofu, which is the type that is typically used more as a meat replacement. It is made by basically pressing soy milk into a block. Tofu has a bland taste, but that makes it ideal for seasoning however you like.

Tofu is an excellent source of protein and does contain the nine essential amino acids, which are important for muscle health. It also provides a good source of iron and calcium, making it beneficial for maintaining healthy bones and decreasing the risk for osteoporosis.

Tofu can actually lower your bad cholesterol and decrease the risk for heart disease. It may also prevent certain cancers such as prostate and colon. Due to its high protein and fiber content, tofu may help you feel full longer and help you control your weight as well.

Some people are concerned about the effects of eating soy, particularly people who have survived breast cancer. However, soy or tofu contains plant estrogens, which actually may lower the risk of breast cancer because of the effect of plant estrogen on the human body. It can also be used for menopausal women to help decrease the frequency of hot flashes. This was first noticed in Japanese women, who tend to have milder menopause symptoms than women in other cultures due to their diet. If you take medications for depression (monoamine oxidase inhibitors or MAOIs) or Parkinson's disease, it is suggested that you do not eat tofu due to the risk that it could raise your blood pressure dangerously high.

When using tofu as a meat replacement, you want to use the extra-firm variety. After pressing the water out, you can cook it in a variety of ways, such as sautéed, pan-fried, and grilled. Marinating it first helps to impart even more flavor as well.

Tempeh

Tempeh, also made from soy, is chewier and has a nuttier taste than tofu, but it can still be flavored and seasoned in different ways. Tempeh is very high in iron and is cholesterol-free. It is made by fermenting entire soybeans and pressing them into a cake.

Nutrition-wise, tempeh actually contains vitamin B12, which is sometimes difficult for vegans and vegetarians to get in their diet since it is typically found in animal sources. If you are wondering why tempeh contains vitamin B12 but tofu does not (they both are made from soy), it is due to the fermentation process. Like tofu, tempeh contains all nine of the essential amino acids and offers many of the same health benefits. Tempeh, however, contains more iron per serving than does tofu. Be aware that tempeh can actually be made from other beans, brown rice, and seeds.

Due to its chewy texture, tempeh does need to be steamed to soften it up. It also does well with a marinade and can be cooked in a variety of ways. I have used it as a ground beef replacement in a taco bowl. After cooking it, I placed it in a food processor and processed it until it resembled bits of ground beef. Then I assembled my 100-percent plant-based bowl for a delicious meal.

Seitan

This is my newest discovery, and to say I am obsessed is an understatement! Seitan (pronounced "say-tan") is known as "wheat meat," so it is not ideal for those who have gluten sensitivity, but it is a wonderful meat replacement for everyone else due to its meat-like texture.

Seitan is sold in a variety of forms, such as strips or slices. It is made by rinsing away the starch from dough that is made from wheat, leaving behind the high-protein form. It too can take on many different flavors and on its own has a savory taste. Some describe it as similar to bland chicken or even a portobello mushroom. I made **BBQ Ribz** using seitan and it was delicious! It was like eating a plate of boneless ribs, and they were drizzled in my homemade **Tablespoon BBQ sauce**. The next cookout I go to, I will definitely be taking a plate of these with my favorite side dish for a delicious combo.

Other Plant-Based Meat Replacements

These are appearing on menus in restaurants throughout the country. The Beyond Burger, Impossible Burger, and other plant-based burger substitutes add another option for meat replacement. However, I do urge caution because these meat replacements—although they may have no cholesterol—are high in sodium and saturated fat. Also, the jury is still out on the long-term effects of the pigments that are used to color them to make them look like meat. The plant-based meat replacement that I prefer is sold at Trader Joe's. It is called Beef-less Ground Beef and has a much healthier profile than the products mentioned above. I would just caution that if you are going to eat these, do so in moderation—or you could just use tempeh or seitan instead as a ground beef replacement.

W FOR WATER

No list of healthy, must-have foods would be complete without water. Whatever you may call it, water, *agua*, or H_2O, it does a body good! The average adult human body is 50–65 percent water. Your brain, heart, lungs, and even bones all contain varying amounts of water.

Water has a multitude of health benefits, so I will list just a few here:

- Acts as a shock absorber for the brain and spinal cord.
- Plays an important role in maintaining healthy joints.
- Helps to flush waste from your body in the form of urine made by the kidneys.
- Helps regulate bowel movements and prevent constipation.
- Helps to control body temperature when you sweat.
- Helps improve skin complexion.
- Lubricates joints.

- Makes saliva, which prevents dry mouth.
- Prevents and treats headaches.
- Helps your brain work better and improves mood and concentration.
- Helps with weight loss.

When you hydrate properly, you help all the major organs of your body function better. You also can help control your weight with water because when you drink water before a meal, you are less likely to overeat at a meal and also less likely to snack in between meals. Being dehydrated can make you feel sluggish and fatigued and can cause muscle aches as well.

So just how much water do you need to drink each day? We often mistake thirst for hunger and eat instead of drinking water. What we don't realize is that by the time we recognize that we are thirsty, we are probably already 10 percent dehydrated. Every part of your body benefits from being well-hydrated, from your brain to the muscles in your feet. Aim for 11½ cups a day for women and 15½ cups a day for men. You may need more or less depending on your personal exercise levels and health issues, so be sure to check with your doctor. Keep in mind that you can also get water through food sources as well, such as fruits and vegetables that have high water contents. These include watermelons (and other melons), strawberries, tomatoes, apples, zucchinis, bell peppers, and oranges, just to name a few. High water content is why it is important to sauté your bell peppers *before* adding them to dishes like meatloaf to prevent creating a dish with too much water content (take it from me). Coffee and tea are also high in water content and contain beneficial antioxidants.

A common complaint people have is that water is so bland and that is why they do not drink as much as they should. One way around this is to add items to it such as lemons, ginger, and basil. I use these in my recipe for flavored water. By doing so, you increase the antioxidant, anti-inflammatory, and disease-fighting properties while staying hydrated. Other options include oranges, limes, berries, cucumbers, and fresh herbs. You can also set reminders throughout the day that help you to drink more water, such as setting alarms on your watch or using water bottles that are marked with positive reinforcements to drink a certain amount of water per hour.

My **Lemon, Ginger, and Basil Water** recipe is simple and refreshing. Add some frozen pieces of fruit for a colorful and flavorful thirst quencher.

X FOR EXTRA VIRGIN OLIVE OIL

Okay, so I stretched a bit here, but can you blame me? Surely I do not have to explain why I have included it on my favorites list. Extra virgin olive oil (EVOO) is pretty much everywhere you look, and with good reason, because its mild flavor pairs well with so many different things (balsamic vinegar, I'm looking at you), and it can be used in anything from appetizers to dessert. In fact, many Italian restaurants offer olive oil with balsamic vinegar instead of butter with their delicious warm and crusty bread.

Let's look at just a few of the many health benefits of EVOO:

- Rich in the good types of fat. Olive oil is made from olives, and it contains mostly monounsaturated fats, which have been shown to decrease inflammation and may even decrease cancer. Monounsaturated fats decrease LDL cholesterol, the cholesterol that clogs arteries and leads to stroke and heart attacks.
- Contains the antioxidant vitamin E, which also helps fight inflammation. Inflammation increases the risk for chronic diseases such as Alzheimer's disease, heart disease, stroke, and diabetes.
- Contains vitamin K, which helps your blood to clot normally and strengthens bones by controlling how calcium gets deposited in your bones.
- Despite being all fat, EVOO is not typically associated with weight gain when used in small amounts. One tablespoon of EVOO, which is one serving, contains about 120 calories. While this can certainly add up if your recipe calls for 3 tablespoons or ½ cup, keep in mind that you will be eating fractions of that meal you prepared, so the calories will be proportionate to how much you ate at one time. Also, when being used to cook vegetables or in an otherwise low-calorie salad dressing, the net effect will be negligible because the accompanying vegetables are usually low in calories (depending, of course, on what else you add to them #allsaladsarenothealthy).
- Has antibacterial properties.

There are different types of olive oil, such as virgin olive oil, which is less expensive than EVOO, and light olive oil. EVOO is the highest quality and therefore the most expensive. It is made from the first pressing of olives, whereas virgin olive oil comes from the second pressing. My personal favorite thing about EVOO is that it can be used in many different ways to cook. It can be used in place of butter in baking or sautéing vegetables, although this is actually not recommended by some experts due to its smoke point (the temperature at which an oil starts to smoke) and higher price tag. For frying and cooking at higher temperatures, consider using avocado, grapeseed, or peanut oils. EVOO is also a key ingredient in salad dressings and vinaigrettes in a 1:3 ratio (one part vinegar to three parts oil).

While many people (including myself, before I researched this topic) store their EVOO right beside the stove, this is actually not the best thing to do. It is recommended that you store it in a dark bottle or cabinet, away from the heat of your stove. This prevents the oxidation that will turn your oil rancid (*yuck!*). However, I think that if you use your EVOO often (like I do), it will not have time to turn rancid. Just don't buy large quantities of it at one time if you will not be using it that often.

My **Vegan Green Goddess Dressing** uses EVOO and a *bunch* of green vegetables and herbs, including tarragon, chives, spinach, cilantro, avocados, and scallions. It was a collaboration between my mom and me, and I think we did a pretty delicious job!

Y FOR NUTRITIONAL YEAST

This is another new find for me, and now I *cannot* imagine life without it! I mean, how can you go wrong with something that literally has the word *nutritional* in its name? We will get to the health benefits in a minute, but seriously people, this stuff is amazing! Nutritional yeast adds a cheesy, savory flavor to dishes such as mac 'n' cheese, popcorn, pizza, baked potatoes, soups, scrambled eggs, and tofu, just to name a few. And the timing of this discovery could not have been more perfect: nutritional yeast appeared just in time to make it onto my **Favorite Vegan Foods ABCs** list for the letter Y. Of course, I *had* to use nutritional yeast to make a creamy, cheesy vegan mac 'n' cheese recipe. I looked up a lot of vegan mac 'n' cheese recipes but was unable to find one with both nutritional yeast and store-bought vegan cheddar cheese. So, I did what any good Physician In The Kitchen would do: I went to the lab and created my own! I used both the nutritional yeast and vegan cheddar cheese to bump up the cheesy flavor and gooey-ness, because those are *not* negotiable when it comes to mac 'n' cheese. Giving this classic comfort food a healthy makeover was a tad stressful because mac 'n' cheese is so iconic and well-loved, but I am so happy with the outcome.

But before I share this earth-shifting recipe, let's talk about why nutritional yeast made my list. First of all, nutritional yeast is the same type of yeast that is used to make bread and beer, but it is processed differently. It is not active like the yeast you use to make bread. It is soy-free, gluten-free, and sugar-free. It is an excellent source of protein, fiber, vitamins, and minerals. One important nutrient that some brands of nutritional yeast have is vitamin B12. Fortified nutritional yeast contains this vitamin that is typically found in animal sources and can be difficult for some vegans to get in adequate amounts. Other plant sources that contain B12 are mushrooms, tempeh, fortified plant milks, and fortified breakfast cereals. B12 is important for keeping our DNA and nervous systems healthy. It also helps with the production of red blood cells, which carry oxygen all around your body.

Nutritional yeast is a complete protein because it contains all nine of the essential amino acids your body needs to get from food since we cannot make them (quinoa is also a complete protein). These proteins are important in repairing and strengthening muscles.

A few other health highlights about nutritional yeast:

- Contains fiber that helps prevent heart disease by lowering cholesterol and may help control blood sugars.
- Contains antioxidants that help boost your immune system and lower your cancer risk.
- Helps improve recovery after exercising.
- Contains many of the B vitamins besides B12 (folic acid, niacin, riboflavin, thiamine, and B6). B vitamins play many roles in your body, including creating energy, keeping your brain healthy, and regulating cell growth.
- Contains small amounts of minerals like zinc, selenium, iron, calcium, and potassium, which help with growth, heart function, and immune function.
- Does not contain MSG but instead has something called glutamate (a natural compound), which gives it that umami flavor.

A word of caution: People who have migraines, take certain antidepressants (MAOIs), have a yeast allergy, have inflammatory bowel disease, are diabetic, or who take narcotics for chronic pain should discuss with their doctor if nutritional yeast is appropriate for them to take.

Go ahead and try my **Cheezee Vegan Mac 'N' Cheeze** recipe. You're welcome!

Z FOR ZEST

Well, we have made it to the end of the alphabet, but the journey is truly just beginning. I hope you have enjoyed reading this as much as I have enjoyed putting this list together. Hopefully, I have introduced you to some new foods or helped you see some old favorites in a new light. We close out this list with zest. Yes, I am referring to the zest of citrus fruits, but the word nerd in me can't help but think about the other meaning of zest: *great enthusiasm and energy*. That describes my approach to embracing a plant-based diet, and I hope that came across in this book.

I am going to keep this one short and sweet because I have already discussed some of this content in the orange entry. Citrus zest is the best ingredient you have that you are probably not using (I know because I was once just like you). The zest of lemons, limes, and oranges is packed full of flavor (and yes, health benefits) that will elevate the taste of your food. Believe it or not, the zest actually contains more flavor than the juice of the respective fruits. To get the zest, you need to use a Microplane or the smaller-sized side of a box grater. Be careful not to go all the way down to the white fibrous part (the pith) of the peel. This is bitter and doesn't taste very good.

To recap, citrus fruit zest contains fiber, vitamin C, and other antioxidants. Vitamin C helps the body absorb iron, which is important for people with iron deficiency anemia. Lemon peel has antibacterial properties that are good for oral health. Just like so many of the other foods that I have featured in this series, the benefits of eating zest include lowering your risk for cancer and heart disease and boosting your immune system. Lime zest can reduce the risk for asthma and can help you keep a youthful appearance by protecting the skin against the effects of sun exposure. Orange zest contains fiber, beta-carotene (the precursor to vitamin A), B vitamins, and the mineral calcium. Beta-carotene is the plant chemical that gives sweet potatoes, oranges, and carrots their orange color. Your body converts it to vitamin A and uses it to protect your eyes from eye disease and promote healthy skin and hair.

Before you zest, be sure to wash your fruits very well to remove any residual dirt or pesticides, especially if they are not organic. Do not buy those expensive veggie wash products for sale in your produce aisle. Studies have shown they are not more effective than a simple mixture of water and vinegar.[9] You can make a simple produce wash at home by adding one part white vinegar to three parts water in a spray bottle. Spray to coat the surface of the fruit or vegetable and then rinse with clean water. If they are especially dirty, let them soak for 5–10 minutes in your sink or a bowl.

Citrus zest can be added to a variety of dishes, including appetizers, breakfast, salads, and baked goods. My **Lime Cilantro Dressing** can be added to pasta, salad, or your favorite protein.

I hope this series, as well as the entire book, has been as helpful of a starting point for you as it has for me. Now go forth and create your own nutritious and delicious plant-based meals! Remember: #eatyourcolors and invest in your health one plate at a time!

APPENDIX

DR. MONIQUE'S MUST-HAVE KITCHEN UTENSILS AND GADGETS

As the self-avowed "kitchen gadget junkie," I surely have *waaaay* more than my fair share of kitchen utensils and gadgets. But if you are just beginning your kitchen journey, or simply want to know which doohickeys do what, the following list should help you figure out what you may need to add to your kitchen. Who knows? You just may discover one or two (or five) new favorites. Don't blame me, though, if your gadget drawer or cabinets start to get a little crowded. You can find some of my other faves at kit.co/DrMonique.

This list is not meant to be all-inclusive, and I have grouped them into categories to organize them. If you have a favorite gadget or utensil that didn't make my list, send it to me at physicianinthekitchen@drmoniquemay.com or @physicianinthekitchen on Instagram or Facebook.

GENERAL FOOD PREP: *These gadgets and utensils are the workhorses for any kitchen and lay the foundation for a well-equipped kitchen.*

- **Salad spinner:** used for washing and drying fresh produce, including herbs and leafy greens.
- **Strainer/colander:** useful for draining pasta, canned beans, and freshly washed fruit.
- **Measuring cups and spoons (both wet and dry measures):** invaluable for the accurate measuring of small amounts, especially when baking recipes that should be followed as closely as possible (like cakes).
- **Food scale:** useful for portion control and to determine the correct cooking time by weight; get one with different settings like grams, pounds, and fluid ounces.
- **Mixing bowls:** very helpful for efficient cooking, they allow you to have ingredients ready to add quickly during the cooking process. Invest in a few different sizes, and consider whether you want glass, metal, or plastic. I keep one handy during food prep to collect my trash and make cleanup a breeze.
- **Salt and pepper grinders or mills:** for freshly ground salt and black pepper that gives a nice finishing touch to salads, soups, or sauces.
- **Cutting board:** these come in different sizes and are made from different materials (wood, plastic, or rubber), and some have grooves around the perimeter to catch liquids or juices to prevent making a mess.

SHARPIES: *These gadgets have sharp edges and should be used with caution.*

- **Vegetable peeler:** handy for peeling vegetables with a tough outer skin, such as squash, potatoes, and carrots.
- **Vegetable chopper:** as a somewhat knife-challenged individual, I *love* this gadget for chopping onions (it spares the tears), celery, bell peppers, and carrots into evenly sized dices.
- **Kitchen shears or scissors:** goes without saying, but it is good to have a kitchen-dedicated pair on hand. I prefer the ones with a detachable hinge so I can take them apart and place them in the silverware rack of my dishwasher for easy cleaning and sterilization.
- **Mandolin:** used for making uniformly-sized slices of firm fruits and vegetables, like potatoes, apples, or radishes. Be sure to use the guard that comes with it to prevent serious hand injury.
- **Grater:** each side of this (usually) four-sided, rectangular-shaped utensil can be used for slicing or grating cheese, garlic, or ginger.

IT'S ELECTRIC! *These gadgets need to be plugged in but shouldn't take up too much countertop space.*

- **Food processor:** makes quick work of making dough, pesto, salsa, vegan mayo, or aioli.
- **Juicer:** small handheld ones are good for adding citrus juice to recipes. Larger countertop ones are good for larger batches of fruit or vegetable juices. Do your research to determine if you want a centrifugal force juicer, masticating juicer, twin gear juicer, or a juice press. In case you are wondering, I have a masticating juicer.
- **Electric can opener:** try to get one that makes the lid edge dull instead of sharp to prevent injury. Taller ones allow you to open larger cans, and some can even reseal the can to prevent waste. Just be sure to place the resealed can in the fridge and not back in the pantry.
- **Immersion blender:** a small handheld blender useful for making soups, smoothies, salad dressings, and homemade mayo or aioli.

BAKING BASICS: *These utensils are used for baking but certainly can be used for other kitchen tasks as well.*

- **Oven and meat thermometers:** a good oven thermometer is essential to help prevent baking disasters. Your oven display panel may say it is the temperature you set it for, but it actually may not have warmed up sufficiently, resulting in underbaked dishes or cakes. A meat thermometer is important to determine if meat is cooked properly, instead of cutting into it to check for doneness and letting out the juices, which then makes the meat dry.
- **Ramekins:** these small ceramic baking dishes are perfect for making individual or one-serving dishes, such as French onion soup, soufflés, or chocolate pudding. Think of them as built-in portion control!
- **Rolling pin:** if you enjoy making bread or pie crusts, this is a must-have for that "made from scratch" seal on your dinner rolls, pies, pizza crusts, or calzones. Choose a lightweight one to prevent hand, wrist, or forearm strain.
- **Flour sifter:** used for sifting flour or confectioners' sugar but can also be used to sort dried beans and lentils and pick out any debris such as stones they may contain.
- **Pastry brush:** used to brush melted butter, aquafaba, or egg wash onto food before baking. I also use mine to coat the bottom of bakeware to prevent food from sticking.

KEEP IT MOVING: *These utensils are used to move food around during preparation or serving.*

- **Spatulas:** made from rubber, silicone, or metal, these flat utensils are useful for mixing wet and dry ingredients together, scraping out bowls and jars so you get every bit of what you have made or bought, and spreading cake batters.
- **Whisks:** used to whip aquafaba or egg yolks, they add air into mixtures and blend ingredients together until smooth like gravy. Can be wire or rubber (I prefer metal).
- **Tongs:** allow you to pick up or move items while they are grilling or cooking and can be used to serve food such as spaghetti or salad.
- **Slotted spoons:** these spoons have slots or holes in them to allow you to remove solid food from your pot or bowl without the excess liquid.
- **Wooden spoons:** good to have on hand to protect certain cookware surfaces such as cast-iron, nonstick, and stainless steel from scratches; great for stirring gravy or sauce.
- **Serving spoons:** when you want to be the "hostess with the mostest," lay out a set of these and give your table or buffet an elegant touch.

References

[1] American Heart Association News, "Saturated Fats: Why All the Hubbub over Coconuts?," Heart Attack and Stroke Symptoms (The American Heart Association, Inc., June 21, 2017), https://www.heart.org/en/news/2018/05/01/saturated-fats-why-all-the-hubbub-over-coconuts.

[2] Michael Greger, "How Not to Die From Breast Cancer," in *How Not to Die* (New York, NY: Flatiron Books, 2015), 195.

[3] Chris Iliades, "Does Cooking in Cast Iron Help Iron Deficiency?," University Health News Daily (University Health News, January 13, 2021), https://universityhealthnews.com/daily/energy-fatigue/use-cast-iron-cookware-as-an-iron-deficiency-treatment/.

[4] Mickey Nguyen, "The Real Reason Why Cilantro Tastes Like Soap," Delishably (Maven Media Brands, LLC, December 19, 2019), https://delishably.com/spices-seasonings/Why-Does-Cilantro-Taste-Bad.

[5] Ricepedia, "Rice as Food," Ricepedia (Rice Almanac), accessed October 15, 2021, https://ricepedia.org/rice-as-food.

[6] Elena Conis, "The hidden salt in chicken," Los Angeles Times (California Times, June 22, 2009), https://www.latimes.com/archives/la-xpm-2009-jun-22-he-nutrition22-story.html.

[7] U.S. Food & Drug Administration, "Sodium In Your Diet," U.S. Food & Drug Administration (United States Government, accessed October 15, 2021, https://www.fda.gov/food/nutrition-education-resources-materials/sodium-your-diet.

[8] Food Network, "Know It All: Salt," (Food Network Magazine, March 2016).

[9] Ayn-Monique Klahre, "Do Vegetable Sprays and Washes Actually Work (Or Are They a Waste of Money)?," kitchn (Apartment Therapy, LLC, May 1, 2019), https://www.thekitchn.com/fruit-vegetable-washes-necessary-256783.

– –

"Meal Planning and Cooking PLR Profit Pack" Private Label Content Source. WOWContentClub.com. Accessed November 20, 2020. https://www.plrcontentsource.com/product-page/meal-planning-and-cooking-private-label-profit-pack.

About the Author

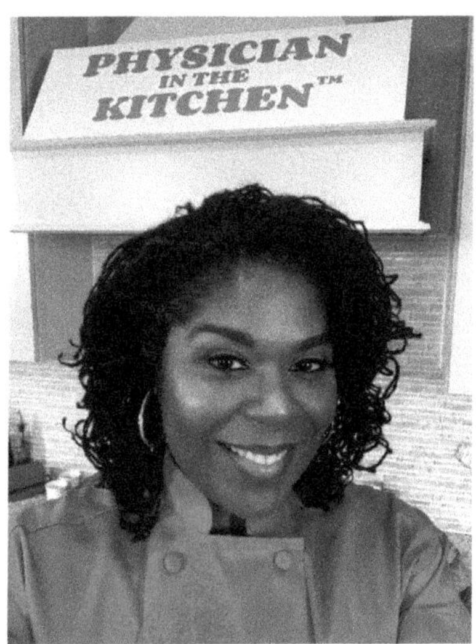

Dr. Monique May, also known as the Physician In The Kitchen®, is the author of the Amazon bestseller, *MealMasters: Your Simple Guide to Modern-Day Meal Planning,* and the founder of Physician in the Kitchen®.

Dr. Monique earned her bachelor of science in psychology at the University of North Carolina at Chapel Hill, and her doctorate of medicine at Temple University School of Medicine with honors. She completed her family practice residency at Carolinas Medical Center, and obtained her master of healthcare administration degree at George Washington University. She is a member of the American Academy of Family Physicians and has received accolades as Resident of the Year in 1999 and Physician of the Year 2019.

Dr. Monique is passionate about using her social platform to educate people on the health benefits of food while showing them ways to save time in the kitchen. She currently resides in Charlotte, North Carolina, with her son, Mitchell.

Learn more at www.drmoniquemay.com

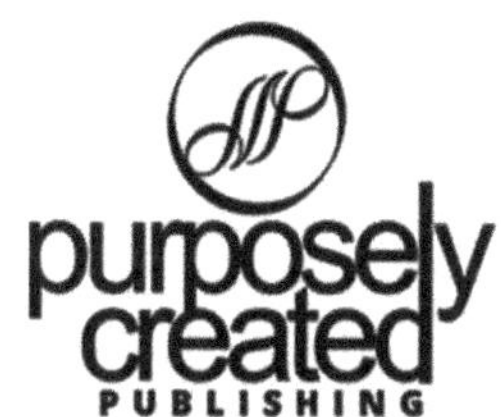

CREATING DISTINCTIVE BOOKS WITH INTENTIONAL RESULTS

We're a collaborative group of creative masterminds with a mission to produce high-quality books to position you for monumental success in the marketplace.

Our professional team of writers, editors, designers, and marketing strategists work closely together to ensure that every detail of your book is a clear representation of the message in your writing.

Want to know more?

Write to us at info@publishyourgift.com
or call (888) 949-6228

Discover great books, exclusive offers, and more at
www.PublishYourGift.com

Connect with us on social media

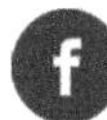  

@publishyourgift